Keto
OVER
50

Simply, fast, tasty diet suggestions on how to prepare everyday healthy-weeknight meals. A new philosophy in healthy living habits to enjoy yourself, your family, your friends, and guests.

PENNY CRAIG

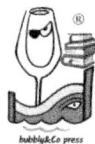

bubbly&Co press

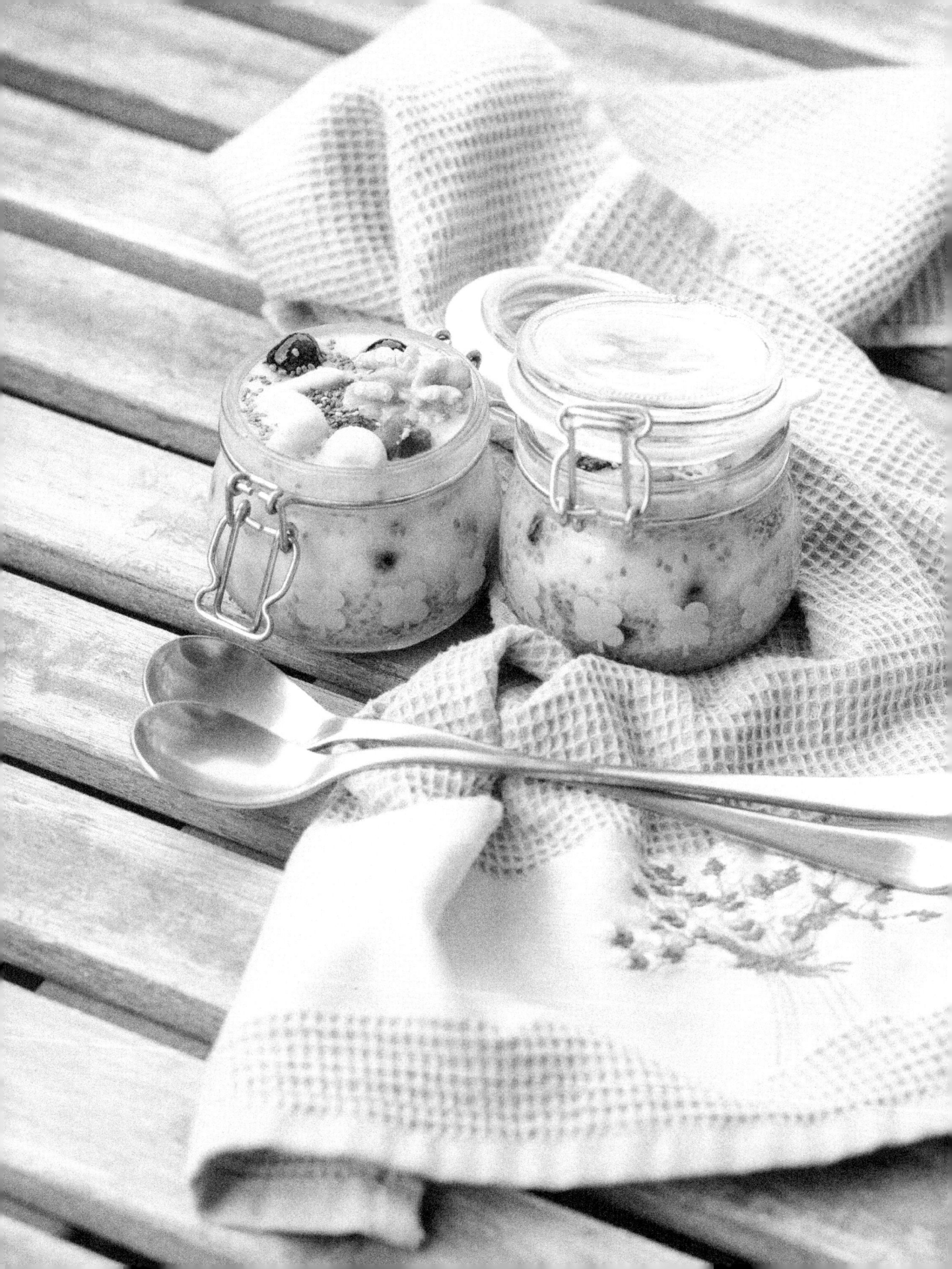

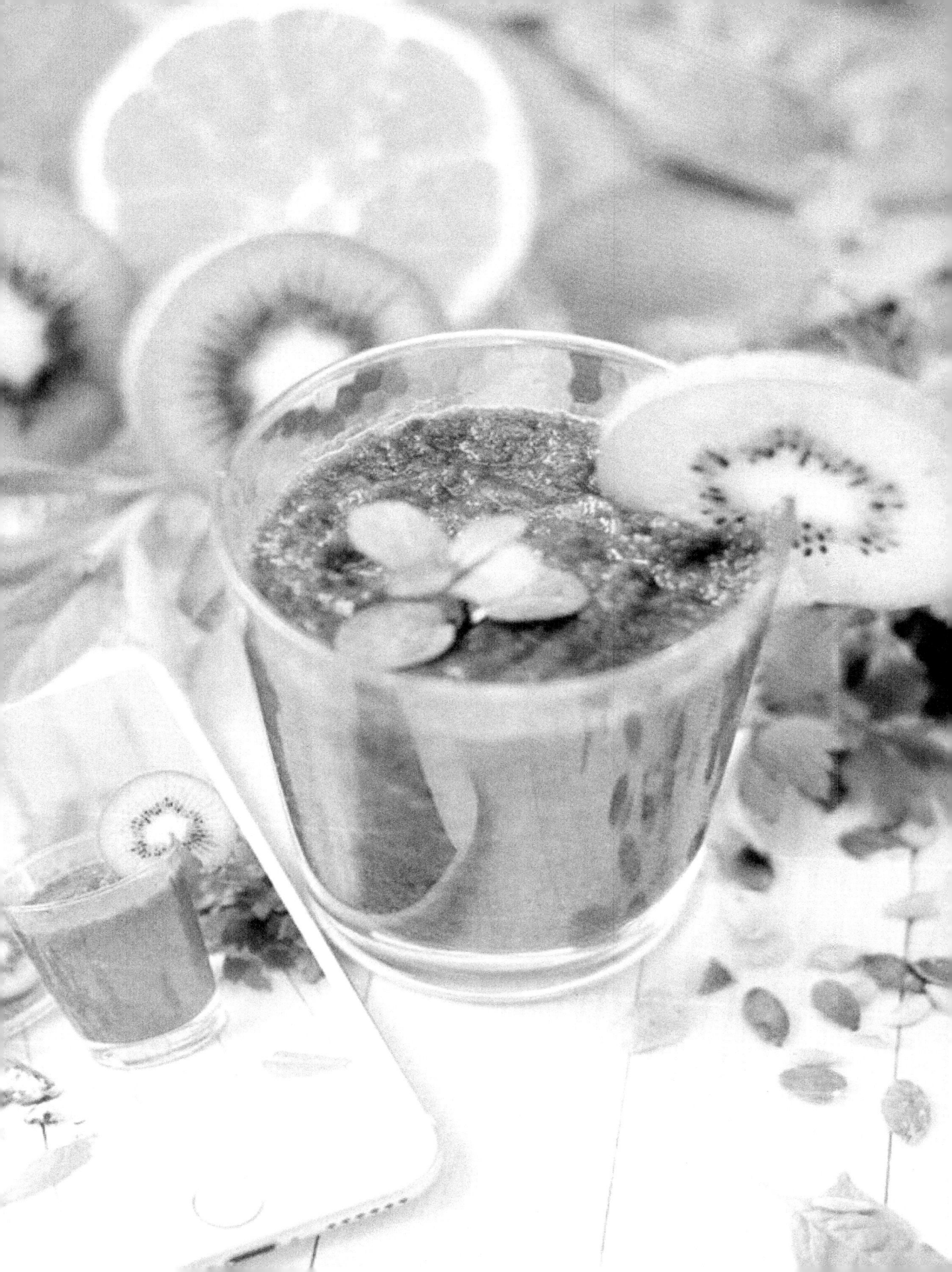

Contents

Introduction

The keto lifestyle is a specific eating plan that revolves around strict adherence to the ketogenic or keto diet. This diet plan has been in use for centuries in one way or another, dating back to the ancient Greeks' time. They were the first to report that the effects of certain diseases and conditions could be lessened, if not cured completely, by following a particular eating plan. One of the conditions they treated with dietary restrictions was epilepsy, known then as "**having fits.**" They noted that people who suffered from "fits" had much less of this if they followed a particular diet.

The twentieth century brought us the first modern study into the effects of diet on "fits," which had been named epilepsy by then. In a small study with a group of patients, doctors found they could restrict the number of seizures per day by having their patients follow a low-calorie, high-fat diet. Since this was before medication had been invented, the doctor's only recourse at the time was to work with a patient's diet and level of activity.

When further looking at the results of the study and trying to determine how it worked so well, scientists discovered that the high-fat diet caused people's bodies to produce three different chemical compounds that were water-soluble and were only found in the bodies of people who were sticking to a starvation diet or one that was high in fat and low in carbohydrates. The scientists called these chemical bodies "**ketone bodies**" thus, the term ketogenic or keto diet was created.

The earliest keto diets were widely varied in the ratio of proteins to fats consumed. The doctors got the idea to try the diet on epilepsy patients, again without using the calorie restrictions. This new plan allowed people to eat until they felt full if their meals consisted of many fats with a moderate amount of protein and low carbohydrates.

The recommendation then was that the carbohydrate intake would not exceed 20 grams per day of all the food a patient ate. This plan reduced the number of seizures, if not eliminating it, but it gave other beneficial side effects. Patients were able to sleep better for longer periods. They lost weight and felt better. Their alertness and attention spans were greatly increased, and children who followed the diet were much better behaved than before.

This diet was widely used as a treatment for **epilepsy** until the middle part of the twentieth century when medications for epilepsy were developed. Swallowing a spoon of liquid or a pill was much easier than following a diet that was so restrictive. It could be difficult to follow the diet if the foods were not readily available. Refrigeration was still not widely available during this time, and many people did not have access to fresh dairy products like milk and cheese. People who lived in the city might not have access to fresh eggs. Much of the population survived on a diet of veggies grown in the home garden and were the staple of the daily diet. As a medical treatment, the keto diet became less widely used until it was no longer taught in medical school and eventually became nothing more than a historical entry in medical history books.

In the nineteen sixties and nineteen seventies, people were very conscious of their appearance, with the newly expanding world of media that gave people access to fashion trends from all around the world. The bikini was the swimsuit all women wanted to wear. The new fad diets also made money as people followed them with guaranteed quick weight loss and a beautiful body.

The keto diet was rediscovered and once again enjoyed popularity. Several different versions were created by different people who touted themselves as experts and named these diets after themselves. But the keto diet came into favor during the nineteen nineties to help a little boy whose seizures were so severe that medicine did not alleviate them. His parents desperately searched for anything that would help their little boy, and they came across medical literature outlining the keto diet and how it was originally used to control epilepsy. The diet was the answer they needed for their son and his seizures. Almost immediately, he stopped having the life-threatening seizures that had plagued him since birth.

So, they made a documentary telling their story, and the keto diet once again jumped into the forefront of popular methods for weight loss. People embraced the keto diet and were fascinated by how it could help them lose weight and improve their lives. Doctors' original studies had recorded notes that most people lost weight and maintained a healthy weight. So, the newest weight-loss sensation was a diet that was originally developed to control seizures in children and adults.

The keto diet basics have been a way of life for our ancestors, who were hunter-gatherers. They gathered whatever fruits and vegetables they could find to supplement their diet's staple, which was the meat they hunted. Our ancestors' diet was heavily based on meat and fat, with an occasional berry or carrot thrown in.

Every generation since then has become more obese as our lifestyles become more sedentary, and our diets become more heavily oriented around carbohydrates. So, what is it about the keto diet that makes it the perfect solution for weight loss and disease prevention? The cause of all these marvelous side effects is a thing known as **ketosis**.

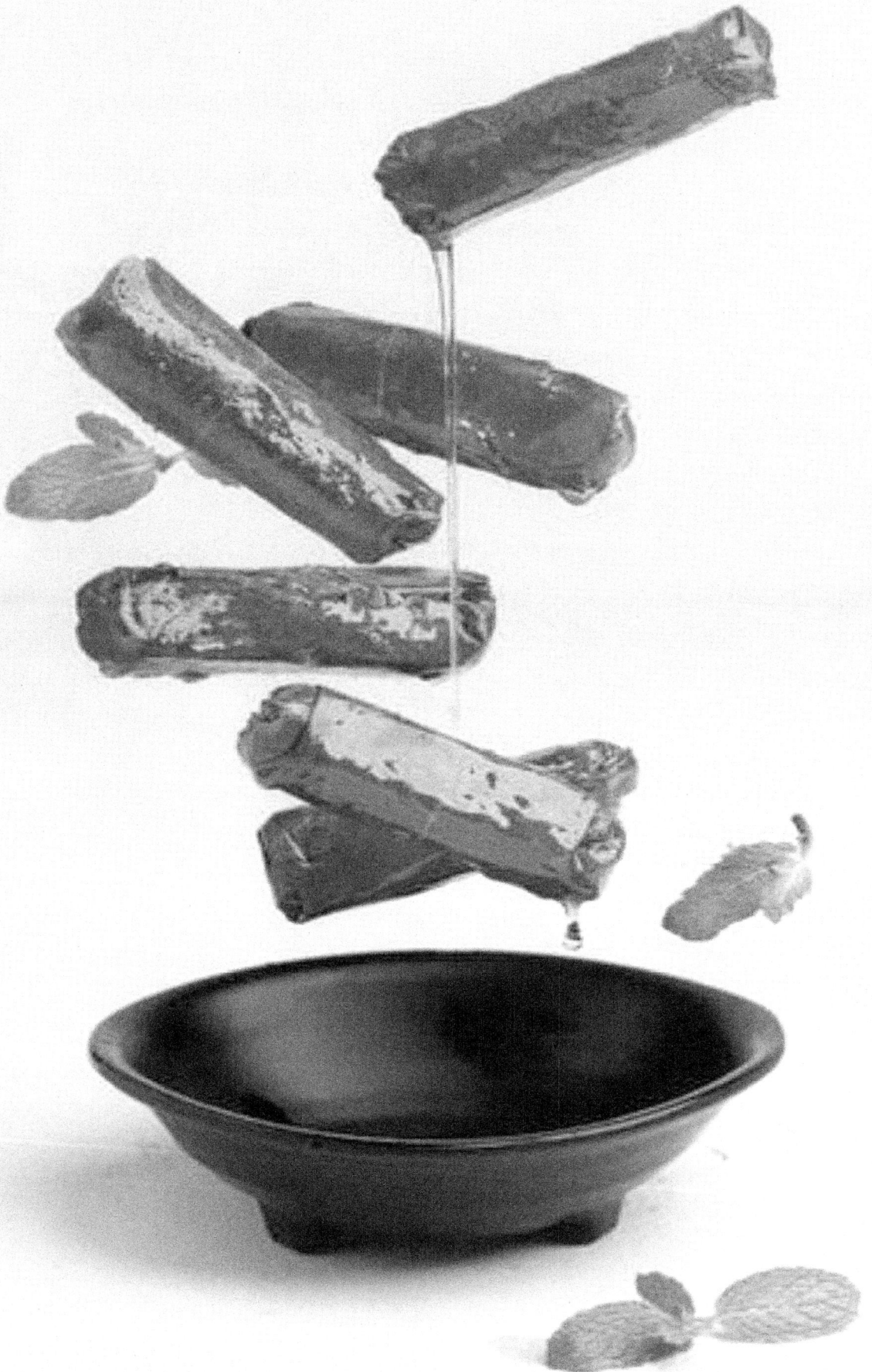

Chapter 1. Keto Simply Concept

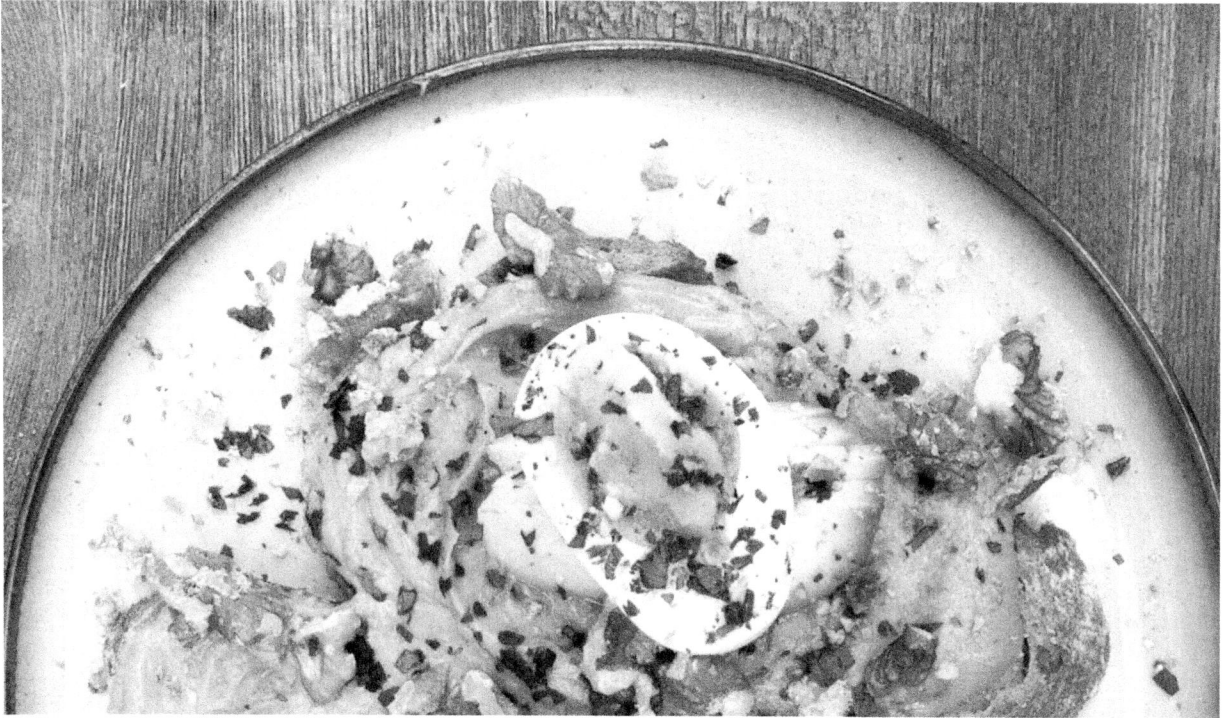

What Is Ketogenic Diet?

Ketogenic diet is a low carbohydrate, high-fat diet that helps people lose weight and fight metabolic disease.+

Most people need at least 20–30 grams of carbs a day to feed their neural networks. However, when you're on a ketogenic diet (or any other kind of low-carb diet) this is not the case. You would be astounded by how many types of vegetables there are that have no more than 5 grams of carbohydrates.

A ketogenic diet is a very low carbohydrate diet consisting of less than 20 carbohydrates per day. Not per meal, yes you read it correctly, per day. It is not for the faint of heart and it is a very challenging way of eating that takes complete dedication. It is not easy, and some people simply find it too restrictive or difficult to maintain. On the flip side, if you are looking to lose weight this way, it can be helpful. If you show up to the ketone diet starving all the time, you won't stick with it.

One of the most important nutrients for fueling our brains is glucose or sugar. The very definition of the Ketogenic Diet is eating a diet that is high in fat and low in carbohydrates (this can also be called low-carb, high fat). When glucose levels are low enough, our bodies start to burn ketones as fuel instead of glucose. When your body is finally in a fat-burning state (ketosis), the level of other key minerals in your body will be affected.

Ketosis is the state in which the body produces ketones in the liver to be used as energy. These are produced from fat (the breakdown of fatty acids), with some help from protein (the synthesis of amino acids). This process usually starts when your insulin levels are low. The body can then break down fats to generate quick energy for the brain cells, muscles, and other organs.

The brain is mostly made of fat, and thus the main problem of any diet that cuts out carbs is how it will supply energy to the brain. Ketones are an ideal source of energy because they have a low rate of oxidation and since they are full of lipids (fat), they don't require a lot of oxygen to fuel them.

Muscles can use ketones as fuel for their rapid metabolism, but this is more difficult since the amount that can be oxidized at once is much smaller than with glucose. Oxidative phosphorylation requires the movement of electrons in a complicated series of chemical reactions which are poorly understood by scientists, but work is underway to create synthetic versions which may be easier for muscles to handle.

The liver, on the other hand, can use ketones for up to 72 hours which means that they do not need to be replaced as often as blood glucose.

What Is Ketosis?

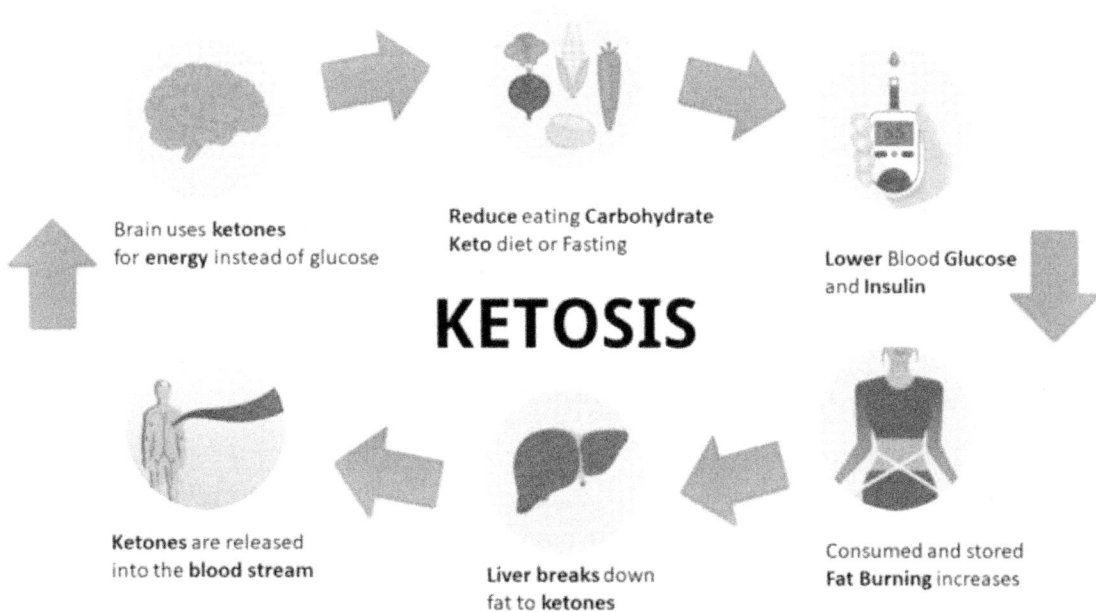

Brain uses **ketones** for **energy** instead of glucose

Reduce eating **Carbohydrate Keto** diet or Fasting

KETOSIS

Lower Blood **Glucose** and **Insulin**

Ketones are released into the **blood stream**

Liver breaks down fat to **ketones**

Consumed and stored **Fat Burning** increases

Ketosis is a metabolic state in humans and other animals, in which some of the body's energy supply comes from ketone bodies in the blood.

Ketosis can be a normal stage of keto-adaptation when your body switches to using fat-based fuels, but it can also be caused by pathogenic conditions such as type 1 diabetes or alcoholism. Dieters greatly appreciate that their brains are fueled well during this process.

The goal of this way of eating is to burn fat and improve your overall health. This diet is widely accepted as one of the most effective ways to lose weight and feel healthier throughout the day (you are less likely to overeat).

The first step to getting into ketosis is to rid your body of any sugar or starch (carbohydrates) you might be consuming.

For this diet to work, you must eliminate all grains, legumes, and fruits (both fresh and dried).

You may also have certain vegetables; however, it is best to stay away from starchy veggies.

If you follow the rules properly, you will get into ketosis within 12–48 hours. Once in ketosis, your body will start using fat as its primary energy source.

Evidence of Ketosis

There is plenty of evidence to support the ketogenic diet, however, it is important to note that there are no official studies that prove its effectiveness.

According to many studies, people on this diet have a much lower risk of developing chronic illnesses, such as type 2 diabetes and heart disease (this is partly because they eat fewer carbs and more fat).

In addition, they claim that you will lose even more weight than you would if you followed traditional methods of eating.

Ketogenic diets may aid in reducing your weight significantly due to their ability to stabilize blood sugar levels. However, they are not just limited to weight loss; a well-regulated ketogenic diet can promote long-term health and wellness by improving insulin sensitivity while also lowering cardiovascular disease risk.

Athletes often use ketogenic diets to increase the availability of energy (in the form of ATP) for endurance-based exercise. They get a massive amount of energy from using fat for fuel. This is the reason why they can perform so well in competitions and why it is seen as such a great method to improve athletic performance.

Ketogenic diets are also useful for certain groups of people. Those who don't feel satisfied when following normal diets may find this way of eating beneficial because it keeps them fuller for longer periods of time.

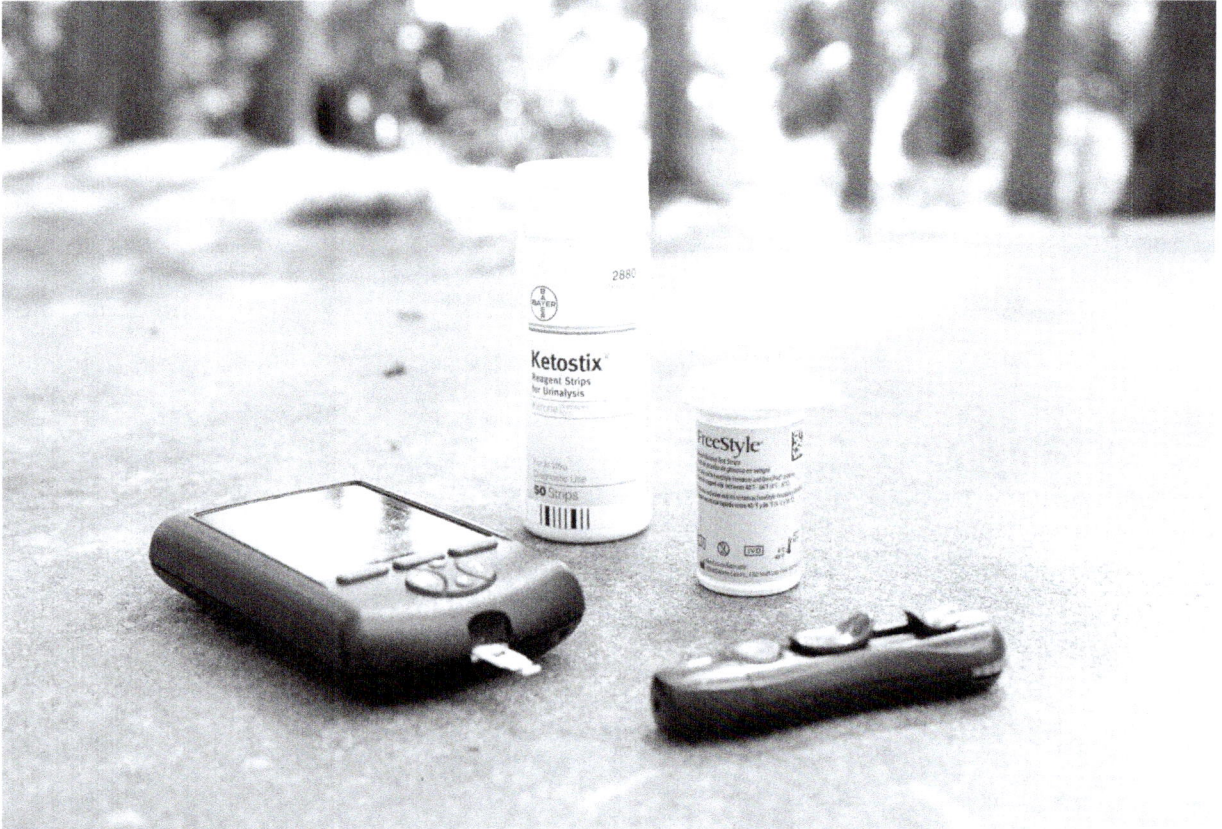

There are a few ways to test for ketosis.

One of the easiest and cheapest ways to determine whether your body is in ketosis is to buy urine testing strips. You can buy them online or in any pharmacy. They will detect the presence of acetoacetate, a ketone body, in your urine.

Once you have determined that you are in ketosis, it is important to know how much fat you should be eating. The standard recommendation is 35% of your daily calories as fat; however, this can be reduced if it causes too many side effects (such as blood sugar issues). This can be determined by using a calorie counter or simply by monitoring your intake.

Many people also believe that they must eat at least 1g of fat per pound they weigh; however, studies have shown that this is not necessarily true. This can be measured with a blood test or by tracking how many calories you are eating and what percentage of calories come from fat (as most foods should contain around 20% of their calories as fat).

Stay away from any diet that restricts carbs unless it is specifically ketogenic, as they are not effective at all.

Examples of Ketosis

The ketogenic diet is used by many people and athletes around the world, from a long-distance runner who consumes fewer than 50 grams of carbohydrates per day to Mike Tyson, who ate 10 eggs every morning to stay strong. It is important that you find what works best for you.

There are many variations on the ketogenic diet which have been created over time. Some are stricter than others and some have special requirements.

Benefits of Ketogenic Diet

There are many benefits of being in a state of ketosis which includes:

- **Reduced inflammation:** A diet that causes the body to use ketone bodies as fuel is known to have benefits to people with inflammatory conditions such as arthritis or other autoimmune disorders. Many have argued that this is because the process of burning fat for fuel helps reduce inflammation and therefore, it may be helpful to those who are at risk.

- **Controls blood glucose levels:** The use of ketone bodies as fuel has been shown to have significant effects on blood glucose levels, especially in diabetics and people who suffer from high blood sugar. This can result in dramatic improvements in energy levels, mood, and insulin regulation.

- **Reduced cravings:** Eating to satiety and avoiding spikes in blood sugar stabilizes insulin levels, which can also improve reasons you might overeat, such as emotional eating or living with a chronic illness.

- **Weight loss:** While it is true that the level of carbohydrates you eat can trigger your weight loss or gain, it is not true that you need to follow a specific diet to lose weight. However, if you are looking for a way to improve your body's ability to burn fat, then this type of diet can certainly help.

- **Improves brain function:** Studies have shown that a keto diet may improve brain function and could be beneficial to those who experience symptoms of Alzheimer's as it may help them to control their blood sugar levels.

- **Decreases risk of chronic illness:** A ketogenic diet has been shown to reduce the risk of developing many chronic illnesses, including cardiovascular disease and type 2 diabetes.

- **Stabilizes blood sugar:** When you are in a state of ketosis, your blood sugar levels become stable. This means that you will have fewer swings in the levels and can therefore avoid the impact of spikes in your blood sugar.

- **Weight maintenance:** Once you reach a weight loss goal or are satisfied with your weight with a ketogenic diet, it is essential to maintain your goal. This can be achieved by consuming additional calories to maintain the same level of metabolism instead of giving in to cravings or falling off the wagon completely.

Most people who follow this type of diet can usually eat whatever they want without feeling nauseous or being "hungry."

How to Get Started with the Keto Diet

There are many ways you can start a ketogenic diet. Remember that you do not need to buy any special food or use special varieties of ingredients. You can eat foods that you are already familiar with and enjoy.

You just need to make sure that you track your macros (the total amount of calories derived from carbohydrates, protein, and fat) and calories consumed to stay within the recommended ratio of fats, proteins, and carbohydrates.

You can currently find several online calculators designed to help you determine your required daily intake of each macro, based on your personal data, to get into ketosis. These tools are very useful for those who are just starting out.

If you want to try this diet out, then keep in mind that it can take a few weeks of trial and error before finding the right balance. If you use the recommended keto calculator, you can make a lot of progress without going too crazy with calorie counting.

To give it a try, start by following this day-by-day meal plan. It is based on eating 100 g of protein, 30 g of fat, and 50 g each of carbohydrates and fiber every day. On top of this base diet (which provides 2,300 calories), there are recommended snacks to consume throughout each day as well as optional foods that will add additional calories. But again, remember that you can alter this diet to meet your specific needs and preferences.

Tips for Success

Be patient, from the first day of starting a ketogenic diet, it may take longer to achieve the results you want, as you will need time to adjust your body's energy systems. The benefits of being in a state of ketosis are generally felt after 4–12 weeks.

Continue to track your macros and calculate volume when calculating calories to avoid going over or under your daily limit. Also, make sure that you know when you last had a certain macronutrient in the body, as some foods will affect how much of each macro they can give.

Deviate as little as necessary from the keto calculator recommended base diet to achieve the results you want. If you follow your macros and stay within the recommended ratio of fats, proteins, and carbohydrates, you will get positive results.

Be prepared to eat slightly more calories than you track daily to maintain your weight. While this may seem like a difficult task at first, it is something that most people can do, especially if they are used to eating out at restaurants. You may also consider using challenges such as eating only food that is high in fiber, fat, or protein for one day or eliminating all carbs for two days. By doing this, you will become more familiar with the types of foods that will fill you up.

Be patient and do not worry if your weight loss is slower than you anticipated. This is a different way of eating, so do not expect the same results as eating a high carbohydrate diet. Focus on making a change that is sustainable for the long term, which means tracking your macros, consuming enough calories to maintain a healthy weight, and enjoying delicious food at the same time.

The keto diet is ideal for those who want to lose weight because it can help you control hunger levels and avoid feeling "hungry." It is also a very effective way of improving health. However, it is not a good choice if you are suffering from hypoglycemia, which means that you will have to follow a strict diet plan and will need to consume more carbohydrates to stabilize blood sugar levels.

While there is an element of starvation involved, once your body adapts its energy source shifts from glucose to fat, so do not worry about eating small meals. On the keto diet, you eat often and regularly.

If you follow these steps, then the keto diet should bring many benefits, including weight loss, better blood glucose control and it may also improve your health.

Side Effects of Ketosis

There are several possible side effects that you may experience if you eat a ketogenic diet. These include:

Constipation

The primary reason why people experience constipation when on this diet is since their fiber intake is very low. You will need to ensure you consume foods high in fiber so that your body can eliminate waste efficiently.

If constipation persists, then consider taking a fiber supplement or using a stool softener.

Bad Breath

Your body will start to release ketones through the process of exhalation, which can contribute to bad breath. You can combat this by consuming foods that promote better oral health, like parsley and peppermint, or by using a tongue scraper.

Bad breath can also be caused by other factors, such as dry mouth, certain medications, or food choices (for example, garlic). Check the list of possible causes before deciding on a method of treatment, which may include brushing teeth after meals and using dental floss daily.

Elevated Uric Acid Levels

Excess uric acid in the body has been linked with heart disease. The uric acid in your body starts to rise when you consume a diet high in carbohydrates, as the highly processed nature of these foods will alter their chemical structure and make them more corrosive than they would be if consumed by themselves. As such, you can reduce your risk of having an elevated uric acid level by eating high-fiber foods. Consume foods that are rich in fiber (fruit and vegetables) and low in added sugars; these will help control your uric acid levels.

Irritability

This is another common side effect experienced during ketosis; however, this may be caused by a few things such as dehydration or too much salt. Make sure that you are drinking enough water and it's not too hot when you consume salt. You can also try adding a pinch of sea salt to a glass of water instead of regular table salt and drink this throughout the day.

If this persists, consider adding some organic lemon juice to your water or rebounding on a mini trampoline. Exercise has been shown to have calming effects on the mind.

Avoiding ketosis side effects is quite easy, so don't worry if you are experiencing one of the above symptoms. Just make sure that you are consuming enough water and that you are not overlooking any other possible reasons for your discomfort beyond the fact that your body is adjusting to ketosis.

Achieving Ketosis

The most important step is ensuring that you are getting all the food groups you need to thrive, especially protein, which is highly recommended for optimal health. If you are following the standard **ketogenic diet** or modified **Atkins diet** (which lasts from 4–8 weeks), your goal, whether you realize it or not, would most likely be to get into a state of ketosis. To do so, you must keep a constant calorie intake during this period and avoid foods high in carbs.

If you can't get into a state of ketosis, you are not eating the right kind of foods to fuel your body. Some people experience this on a cyclical basis, where they would eat a high amount of carbs for a few weeks and achieve ketosis only to be left without any energy or willpower. What often happens here is that people give in to temptation and consume foods containing sugars or junk food, which can make the whole process much harder than it needs to be.

When it comes to achieving ketosis, there are two methods that you can use to do so. **The first** is the targeted ketogenic diet, which is a strict and short-term diet lasting around 5–6 weeks. **The second method** is the slow transition into the diet, where you gradually decrease your carb intake over a period of 10–12 weeks, which allows your body to adapt slowly fully to using ketones instead of glucose for energy.

There are several ways that you can measure whether you are in ketosis. While urine tests and blood tests are most common, they may not be effective in determining the amount of time that it will take for your body to produce enough ketones on its own.

Your best bet is to use blood ketone testing strips that you can buy from the pharmacy. They can be purchased either in-can or hand-held versions. In-can versions are usually more accurate since they are measured directly from the blood without any other interference.

People at high risk of diabetes or heart disease often have a higher need for energy and would benefit from working out to keep their bodies in peak condition. If you are an athlete, you will want to try your best to make these changes so that you stay at the top of your physical condition and perform well both during training and at competitions.

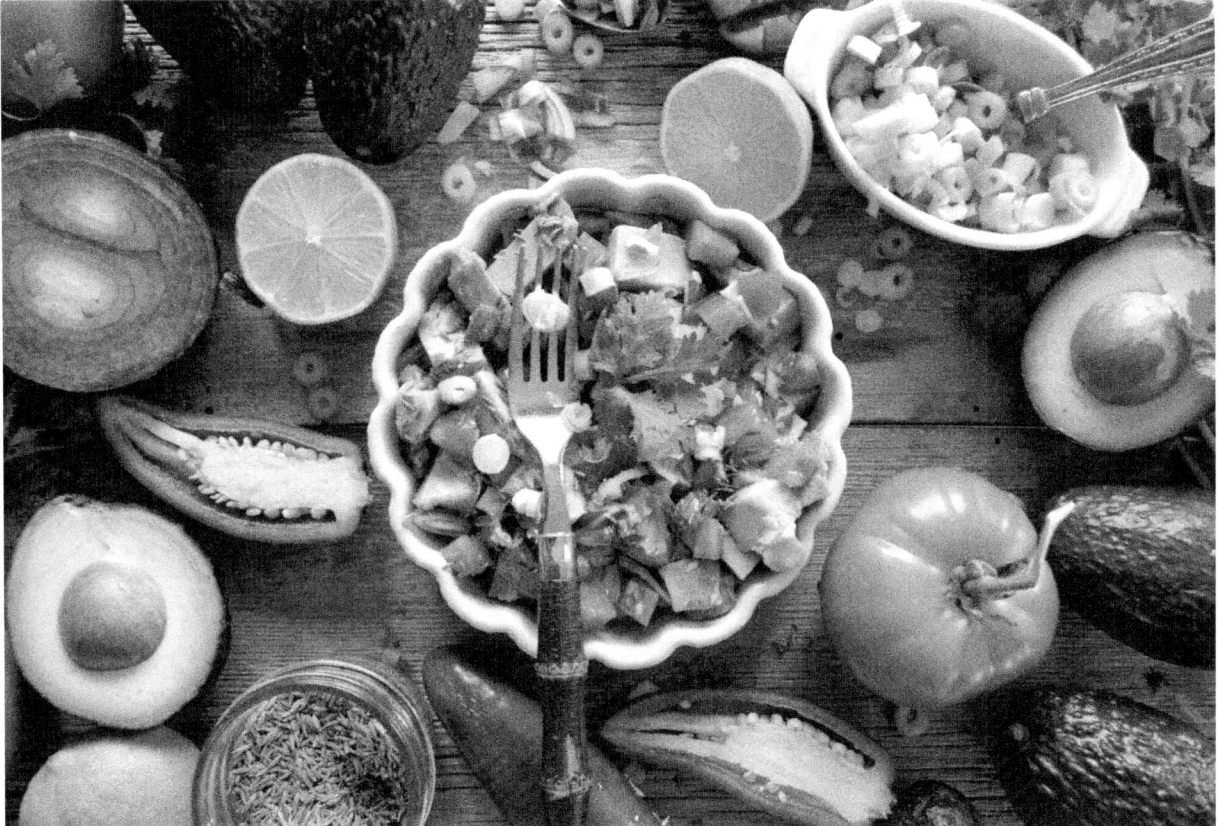

Foods that are high in fat are recommended to eat when you begin the ketogenic diet as they will act as your primary source of energy. As such, your diet should contain:

Fats: These should account for around 70% of your total daily intake. The best sources of fat are avocados, butter, olive oil, and full-fat dairy products. Meats: Meat is an excellent source of protein and contains fat; however, make sure that you buy lean meat instead of junk food products like hotdogs or sausages. These contain high levels of salt and preservatives that aren't needed on this diet, so avoid them entirely.

Fish: Fresh Wild Fish will also be an optimum source of protein and contain omega-3 fatty acids. Omega-3s are incredibly important as they help your brain and nervous system operate properly. The best sources of fish are white cod, mackerel, anchoes', wild tuna, red snapper and salmon.

Eggs: Eggs are an excellent source of protein and contain many other nutrients too. They are a great way to start the day as they provide lots of energy for a long period of time. Look for whole eggs from organic sources where possible as those from chickens raised in warehouses have been shown to have higher levels of cholesterol and hormones that can be harmful to you.

Vegetables: Vegetables contain fiber, which acts as a laxative after eating them. They can be eaten daily or in portions on a weekend. They are also a great source of minerals and vitamins, including potassium, calcium, magnesium, and more.

Healthy Fats

Choose fats that are saturated rather than polyunsaturated ones because trans fats can be bad for your heart. You only need small amounts of saturated fat in your diet as high amounts won't provide you with many benefits.

The best sources of saturated fat are:

- **Coconut oil:** This is a great butter alternative with incredible health benefits and is also very ketogenic, so you can use it in many ways to add extra flavor or nutritional value to your food. It will help with losing weight too; research has shown that it reduces appetite and increases energy by raising metabolic rate.

- **Avocado oil:** This eats like coconut oil, except that it is slightly high in calories, so if you're trying to lose weight, it's not the best choice.
  Sources of trans-fat in each food are highlighted in pink.

Unsaturated fats. When choosing unsaturated fats, look for ones that are monounsaturated rather than polyunsaturated ones (which can be harmful). These include:

- **Extra Virgin Olive Oil:** This is one of the highest quality oils and can be used as part of a healthy keto diet. Evoo is the best type to purchase since it has the most beneficial nutrients and antioxidants.
  Try using Evoo in your cooking, on salads, or as a garlicky dip for veggies. If you can't handle the flavor of this oil, then you can always dilute it with other oils that don't have a strong flavor, such as safflower or sunflower oils.
- **Avocado:** This has been shown to have some great health benefits if you eat it regularly enough, largely because of its high fat and fiber levels.
- **Macadamia:** This is another one that contains high amounts of monounsaturated fats and has a low tendency for producing cholesterol.

Foods to Avoid

Foods to avoid are those that contain "carbohydrates" or sugar, starch, and your main source of food is derived from grains, cereals such as rice or bread, and pasta. Fruits (bananas are okay) are also okay in small amounts. Such as:

- Fruits (except bananas)
- Potatoes
- Corn

So, what's the main point? The ketogenic diet is a diet that burns your body's fat stores as its primary fuel. It is an effective way to lose weight and improve your health and it has many benefits over a calorie-restricted or carbohydrate-restricted diet. To start the ketogenic diet, you need to eat more healthy fats (saturated fats), get moderate amounts of protein from meat, and reduce your carb intake by avoiding all starchy vegetables (potatoes, corn, or other starchy vegetables). You will notice that many of these foods are those that people on a Standard American Diet commonly eat, so you may have to adjust to stick with it.

Foods to Eat on Moderation

- These foods include fresh juice from vegetables such as celery and tomatoes.
- Half of a banana is allowed in the morning.
- A small number of berries (blueberries, raspberries, or strawberries) are also allowed daily.
- A few pieces of dark chocolate (70% or higher) per day are also allowed.
- Alcohol in small amounts is also allowed.

Macronutrients for Keto

The ketogenic diet is the most popular low-carb diet. It involves getting around 10% of calories from carbohydrates, 20% from protein, and more than 70% from fat.

The macronutrients are (proportions out of total calories in the food):

- **Fat:** 70% or more calories
- **Protein:** 20% or more calories
- **Carbohydrates:** 10% or fewer calories

Fewer carbohydrates and higher amounts of fat and protein stimulate the production of ketone bodies in the liver, which is then used as fuel in muscles, and in the brain. This leads to a metabolic state called "ketosis" where your body produces enough energy compounds to sustain itself.

Rules of Ketogenic Diet

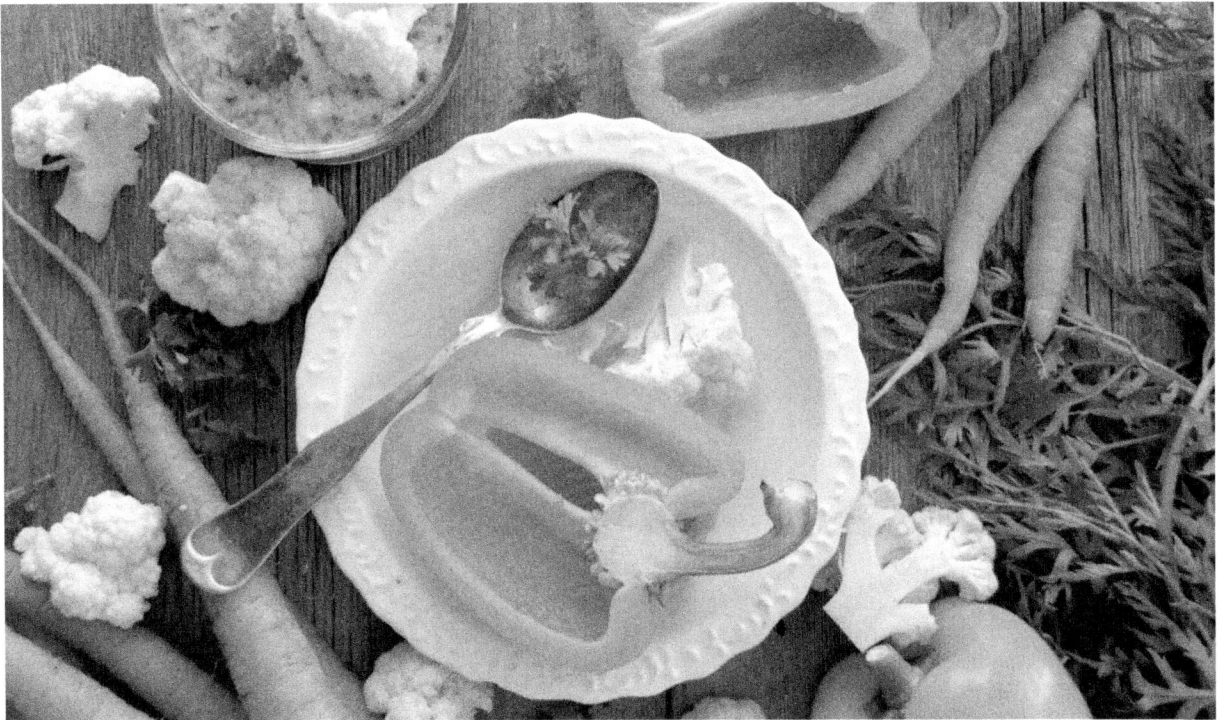

1. **You must stay at 30–60 grams of carbohydrates per day.** But you can have protein in any amount you like. The difference between ketogenic and other diets is that the protein can be almost any type of food, so long as there is no sugar or starch.
2. Starches are low on the restricted list, so be sure to stay away from potatoes, corn, or other starchy veggies and fruits (bananas are okay).

3. Fats are high on the restricted list, so be sure to always include a varied fat source in your diet, such as a wide variety of nuts and seeds (including flax and chia seeds).

4. **You must stay out of sugar and alcohol.** There is no restriction on fat intake so healthy oils (avocado, olives, olive oil, and coconut oil) are allowed as well as lean meat and veggie oils such as olive and flax.

5. You can have wine in moderation with fish, chicken, or beef.

6. **You can increase the amount of protein you eat as you want to keep your protein level high with the goal of staying in ketosis.** But remember that excess protein is converted into glucose which will stop you from getting into ketosis and will make it harder for your body to maintain a fasted state for most of the day, even if you are only sticking with one meal per day.

7. You will need to measure your ketone level with a breathalyzer or use a glucometer to monitor your blood glucose.

8. Drink lots of water and unsweetened tea to make sure you stay hydrated and avoid constipation.

9. **Eat plenty of fat!** You need it to stay in ketosis, so be sure most of your meals are based around healthy fats such as olive oil, flaxseed oil, fish oil, seeds, and nuts such as almonds or walnuts with avocado and coconut for snacks is also good for a high-fat diet as well.

If you follow these rules very closely, you will see the results that you desire.

Meal Prep Tips

You will need to do some meal prep when you start the keto diet. Check out the list of foods allowed or to avoid on the keto diet and you will see that there are a lot of vegetables, healthy fats, meats, and dairy products to include in your daily meals.

Don't forget about your fats! You can throw bacon bits or snack crackers in a storage bag for an easy grab-and-go snack.

The important thing is to continue eating well even when you are not following the keto diet. You need a variety of healthy meals during the day, so you don't get bored with just meat and salad all day long.

Eating keto meals in the morning will keep you full for longer and you can have a variety of food throughout the day.

There are many meals plans that you can follow to help you decide on what foods to eat and how much of each one, but I think it's better to make some basic keto meal prep for your meals and try to stick with them.

When following these basic tips, you won't need much in the way of ingredients. Just some protein (meat, eggs, or fish), carbohydrates from veggies (fresh broccoli, cauliflower, or onion), fat from avocado or salmon, and good fats from coconut oil, olive oil, or flaxseed oil. Cream cheese is a great alternative to sour cream if you don't like using dairy products on your keto diet.

How Much Protein Should I Eat?

When following the keto diet, it's important that you get enough protein in your diet. This can be obtained by eating a variety of meats and dairy, including sardines (my favorite) and cottage cheese (both are high in calcium).

Your body uses the protein you eat to make new muscle and cells as well as the protein that they're using to repair existing muscle tissue. The best way to ensure that you get enough protein is by getting enough food until you have extra energy stores. How much is enough? Your body will tell you how much is needed after 3–4 days. Your exercise level will also determine what number of calories your body needs.

Normal intake of protein should be around 1.5 to 2 grams per kg (1.2 to 1.7 grams per pound) body weight, so you will need to calculate your protein intake when following the keto diet plan. To do this, you'll need to know how many calories your body requires for each day from the Keto Calculator.

A good rule of thumb is that you should eat 0.8 grams of protein per pound of lean mass (body weight/fat). This number is determined by subtracting your body fat percentage from 100% and multiplying by 0.8 (or divide by 4 if you weigh 200 pounds).

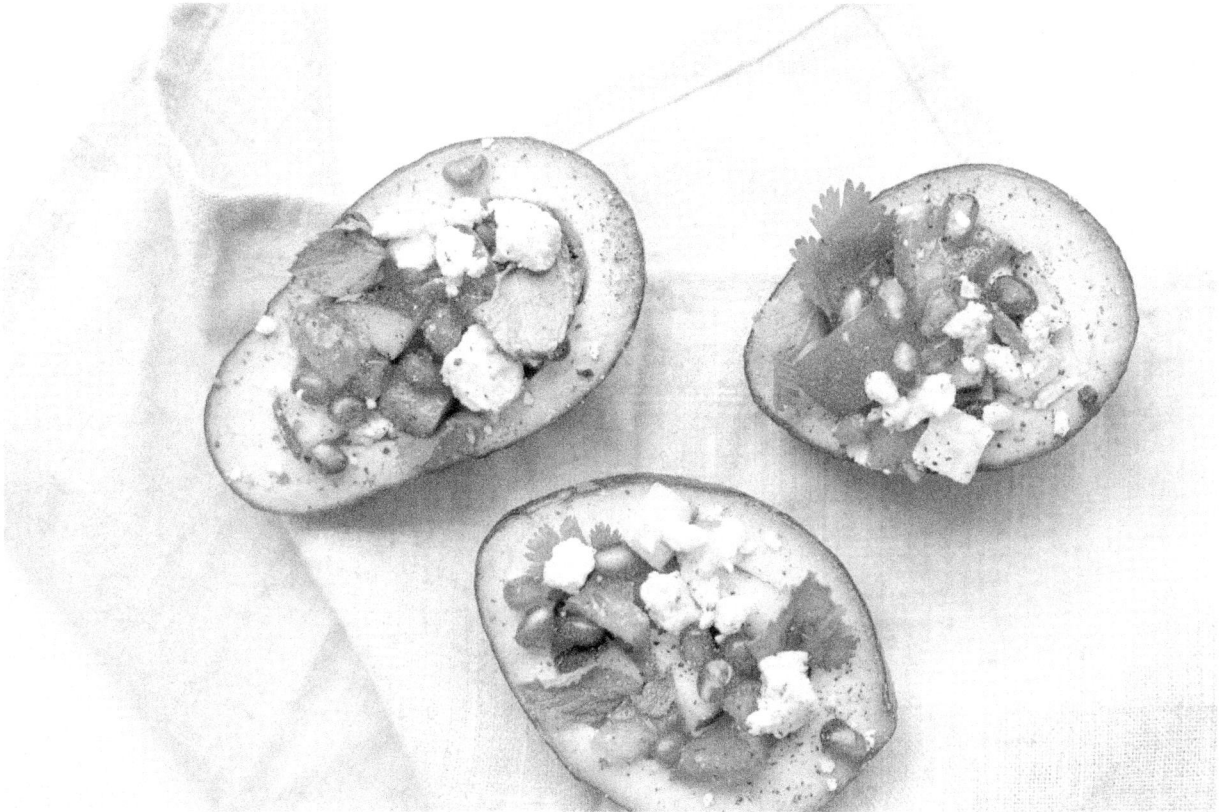

Leftovers are a great thing. You can use them to make delicious low-carb recipes like baked chicken, low-carb soups and salads, chili, or even as a meal on your own. However, not all leftovers will end up in your mouth and you may have to be creative when it comes to making sure that they don't go to waste.

Here are some ideas for dealing with the leftovers from your meals:

- **Understand that they can be used for 3–5 days.** If you want to store them for longer, then freeze them in small portions (you can use these in wraps or simply cut them up and keep them frozen until it's time for another meal).

- **Be creative!** You can make a completely new meal from leftovers or add them to your keto meal plan.

- Try using them in different recipes such as soups, salads, casseroles, frying with other foods if you cook a lot, and many others.

- Throw them in the fridge and start eating them when they've cooled down (this will reduce bacterial growth).

- When I make a recipe that I know will be full of leftovers, I usually make twice the amount to freeze some of it for later. Also, if the meal was cooked in large quantities, then just store it in smaller amounts until you're ready to eat it.

Chapter 2. Body and Mind Changing Over 50

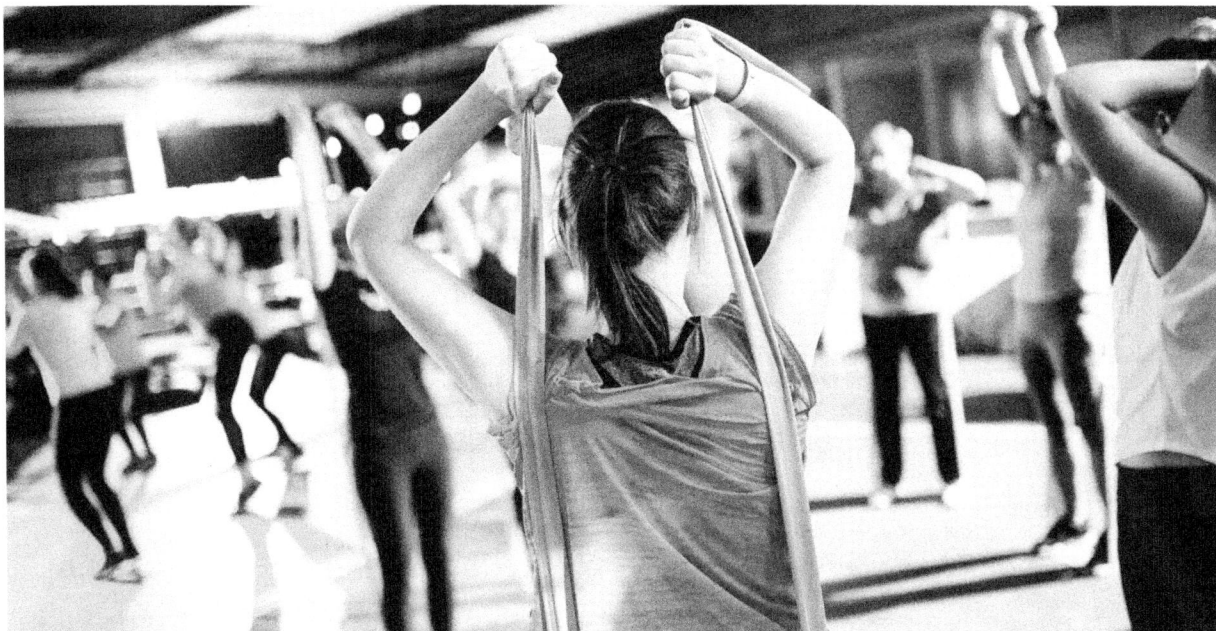

Here, you will learn about many different aspects of the body and mind changing trough the age. It is a time where there are numerous changes happening in your body and your brain. This includes changes to cognitive abilities, behavior, physical function, body composition, etc.

Changes to Body After 50

Although you may not be a teenager or in your twenties anymore, this is a time where it is important to stay active and keep good habits. After 50, it is very important to continue exercising since it keeps the body strong and active. This includes running, weightlifting, walking, etc. However, there are many different exercises that you can do at 50 that you could not do when you were younger. For example, if you're still using weights as a form of training at this age, then there are ways to lift without causing injury or hurting your back. You can focus on your core strength by doing an exercise such as the plie or even walking on an incline. These are just some examples of the exercises you could be doing after 50 to keep your body healthy and strong. Another way to keep the body fit and active is through diet. It is important to eat healthy foods that are good for the body. For example, eating things such as fruits, vegetables, fish, and other lean meats help keep your bones and muscles strong. Also, staying active may increase your appetite, which may affect the foods you eat. Eating more often throughout the day can help with this problem since it keeps you from feeling hungry so often.

Here are common changes to the body after 50:

Weight Gain

When you are over 50, you may experience changes in your weight. Sometimes this is since you are eating more and still staying active. Either way, it is important to remember that this is natural and should not be a cause for concern. If your BMI is staying between 20 and 25 then you are considered healthy.

Menopause

This can occur at any time after 45 years of age in women. However, the average age where it occurs is 51 years old. This change involves a large decrease in estrogen levels which can cause symptoms such as hot flashes, night sweats, mood swings, and much more.

Poor Hearing

This can be caused by the aging process, but this is more common in older men. Also, if you are a smoker, then this may occur faster for you since your hearing is affected by the harmful chemicals in cigarettes.

Smell and Taste Changes

For many people, their sense of smell begins to decrease after 50 years of age. This can be caused by the loss of neurons. The decrease of smell causes problems with food tastes and even other senses such as vision and hearing.

Bone and Muscle Loss

As you get older, it is very common for there to be a decline in bone mass and muscle mass with aging. This is called sarcopenia. This is a normal process that happens with aging, however; it can cause major health problems.

Healthy Weight

If you are overweight and have a BMI of 30 or higher than this may be a cause for concern since it can lead to many other health-related problems. Also, obese individuals tend to have higher risks for heart disease, stroke, diabetes, and even certain types of cancer.

Skin Wrinkles

Unfortunately, as we age, the skin begins to lose collagen and the elasticity in our skin begins to fade. The result is wrinkles and sagging of the skin. In addition, you may notice that your skin either appears pale or ashen, depending on the amount of blood flow to that area.

Joint and Muscle Pain

As we age, there are many changes in the body that can affect joints. The joints begin to weaken, and this can cause pain throughout the body. This is often noticed in the knees, ankles, and back since these are some of the most used areas in our bodies. Also, this is one of the leading causes of disability in older adults.

Osteoporosis

Women are more likely to have osteoporosis than men overall. Osteoporosis occurs when there is a decrease in bone mass and strength due to aging. This can lead to weak bones which can be very dangerous if there is a fall or other accident.

Changes to Mind After 50

Along with changes taking place in the body and the body's ability to function, there are also many changes that take place in the brain. These changes are called cognitive functions. It is important to understand that this is a normal part of aging and often occurs within individuals due to illnesses or injuries. However, there are things you can do to make sure your memory stays sharp!

Memory Loss

As we age, our memory begins to decline. The hippocampus region of the brain starts to shrink and deteriorate over time. This causes trouble with storing memories as well as processing new ones.

Memory loss can occur for various reasons, including anxiety, depression, high cholesterol, and many other health conditions. It is very common that these issues will cause forgetfulness for a person since the hippocampus is the main memory area in the brain.

Smells

This may not seem like a big deal, but people who are over 50 often have difficulty remembering certain kinds of smells. This happens because the part of our brain that processes these types of smells is starting to go downhill due to aging. Many people have great memories for colors, tastes, or other senses, however; they cannot remember smells at all. This tends to cause some problems with an individual's social interactions in general.

Hearing Problems

As we age, hearing loss can become a major problem. The hearing senses are a huge part of our ability to function. As we get older, these senses start to diminish in the brain so that we cannot hear as well as we can before. Many people will develop this problem with age regardless of whether they have an ear infection or not.

Dementia

This is another problem that occurs naturally with the aging process. It is caused by the deterioration of brain cells and by the loss of blood vessels (called "vascular dementia"). This is the most common type of dementia that older adults can get. It can also be a major problem for a person's overall health and can cause serious issues with behavior.

Vision Changes

It is common for older adults to have problems with their vision due to aging changes. These changes are common and often occur within people who already have an eye problem, like glaucoma. Many people will experience night blindness or the inability to see clearly in dim lighting as well as trouble focusing on objects that are far away from them.

Decline in Cognitive Function

The decline of cognitive function is not only caused by the aging process, but also by many other factors such as depression, stroke, and certain illnesses. This is an issue that focuses on specific areas of the brain, including memory, reasoning, and many different areas. It is also common among individuals with mental illnesses such as schizophrenia.

Mental Health Changes

It is very common for older adults to experience depression and other mental health problems as they age. This means that they are not able to function at their peak level due to these issues which will greatly impact their ability to work and live normally. Organizations such as the Alzheimer's Foundation can be a great resource for helping individuals understand the issues they face and come up with plans to combat them.

Sleep Changes

As we age, we tend to have difficulty sleeping in general. This is since the body naturally loses the ability to sleep as well as it did when we were younger. This means that there will be a decrease in energy and alertness throughout the day because of this change. It is common to have problems falling asleep at night as well and even staying asleep through the night.

Due to aging, drowsiness can become a major problem. It is common for mature adults to have difficulty staying awake during activities or during the day in general. This can cause serious issues for individuals who drive, walk, or do other activities that require alertness.

Training Your Muscles

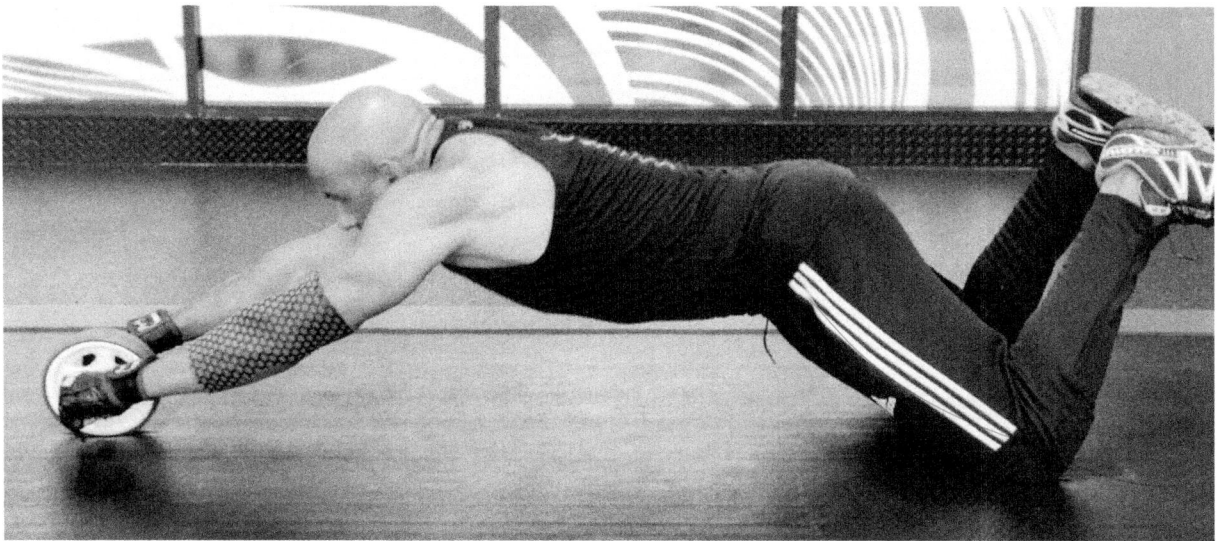

One of the first changes you will notice in your body after 50 is that your muscle mass will start to deteriorate. This means that you will lose muscle mass and strength along with it. In addition to this, there are many other changes that happen in the body, such as the bones starting to break down.

Various conditions can also cause a person to have trouble with their muscles such as arthritis or fibromyalgia. To combat these issues, it is important for individuals to exercise and get their blood flowing within the muscles. This will help increase blood flow and keep the muscles contracted so they do not get weak. Here are some exercises you can try!

Pushups

This is a great way to get a lot of blood in your muscles and strengthen them up. It is best to start out slowly with only 5 or 10 pushups the first time and then increase as you get used to it. Make sure you do some arm stretches before you begin!

Cardio

This is one of the best exercises for getting the blood flowing through your whole body. A great way to do cardio is by taking fast walks outside to get your heart rate up. This will help the muscles stay strong and fight off illnesses that could break them down.

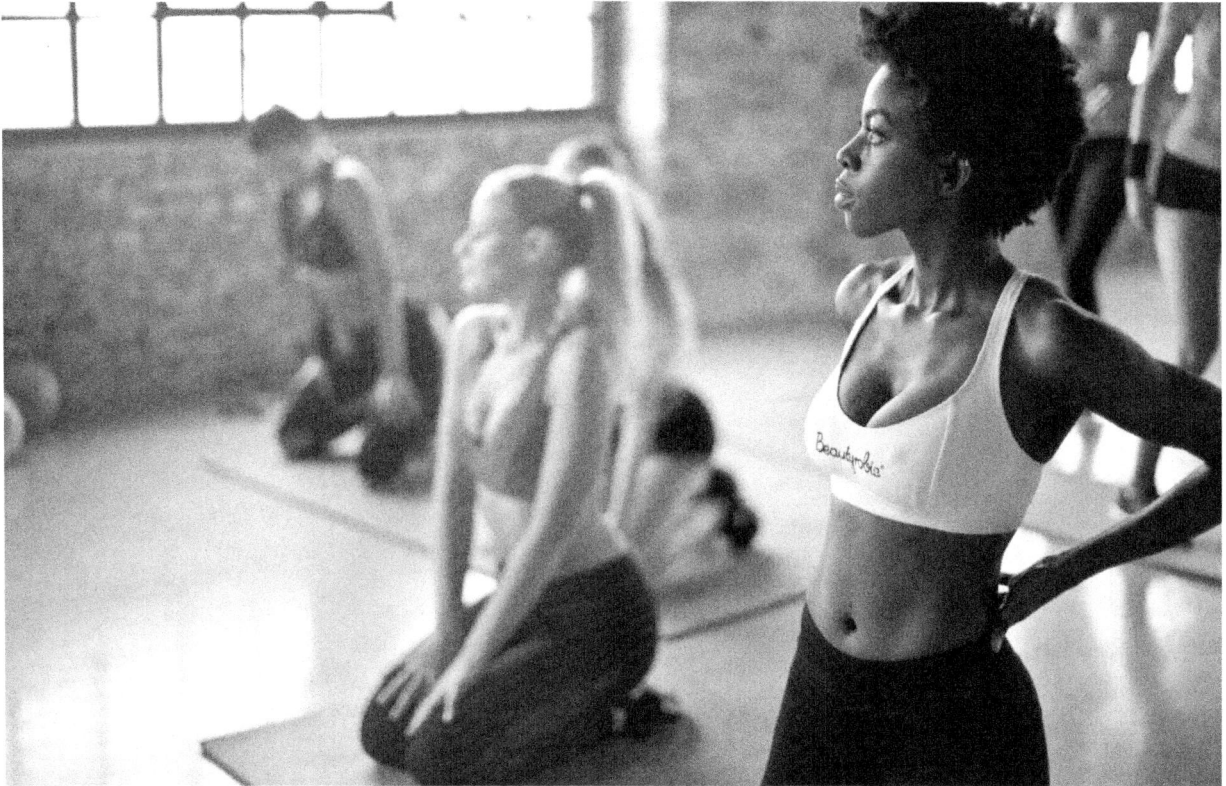

Stretching is also a great way to get your muscles prepped for exercise. You can do this before and after exercising and in the morning to get ready for the day. Stretching will help keep your muscles in good shape and you will have more flexibility in your joints.

Fast Walking

This is a great exercise for all ages! It is a wonderful cardiovascular workout that promotes blood flow and healing of the entire body. You can be as active as you want, but it is best to keep your speed between about 5–7 mph. Try to walk for at least 60 minutes each day, 3–4 times a week.

Swimming

Swimming is another excellent form of cardio that can be done easily. It may take some time to learn how to do it correctly but there are many different swimming styles to explore. You can also try taking classes at your local gym or fitness center if it would benefit you more.

Yoga

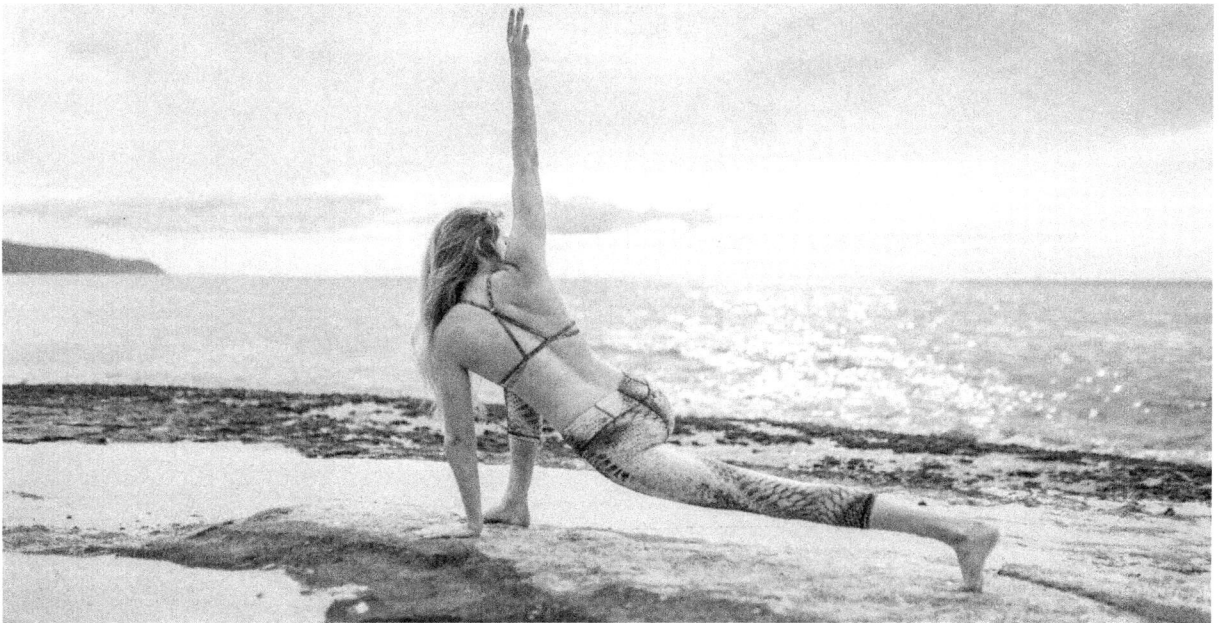

This is a great way to get all your muscles moving at once. It helps strengthen many different areas of the body and allows you to increase flexibility in joints. This is a wonderful workout for anyone.

Choosing a Healthy Diet

Wellness means that is important to eat healthy. Good Diet plan helps with vitamin and nutrient intake as well as helping to fight off any illnesses the body might get. This will also help fight off any weight gain that may come with age.

There are many different factors that go into dietary changes within older adults. Many people will transition out of being heavy meat eaters and start focusing on plant-based foods. There are many reasons for this, including health benefits as well as the environmental impact of eating a lot of meat.

In addition to this, it is also common for older adults to focus more on eating natural foods that do not have additives or excessive ingredients in them. This can help fight off any illnesses that they might be experiencing.

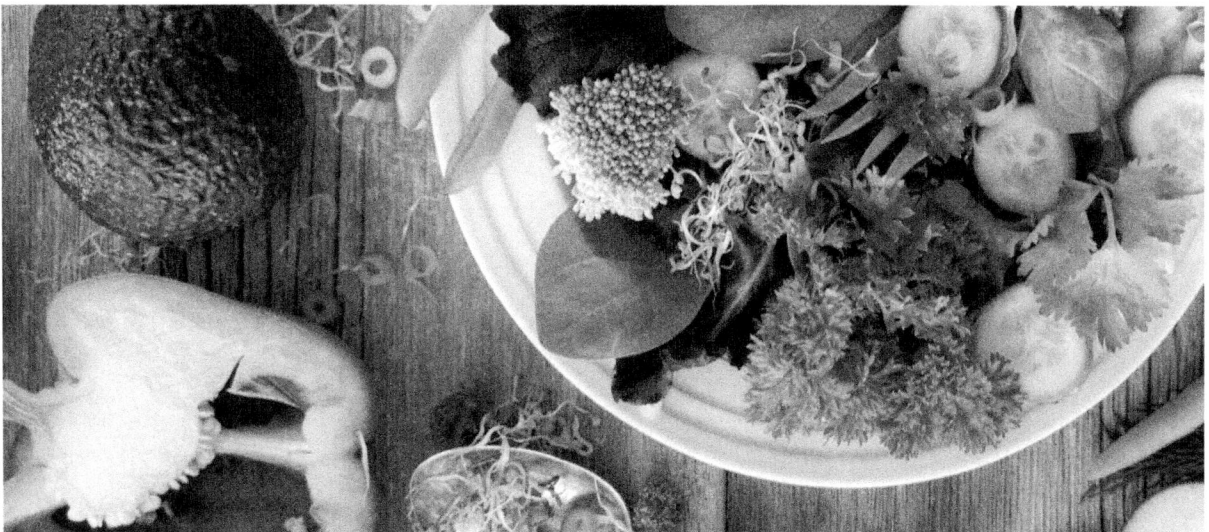

Limit Processed Foods and Junk Food as Much as Possible

Processed foods are full of sugar, salt, oil, and chemicals. This is the perfect food for an older child but not for older adults who are starting to get unhealthy. There are many different natural alternatives to products that do the same job as junk food, such as kelp noodles, lentils, and soy.

Limit Alcohol and Sugars

Older adults should be careful about their alcohol consumption. As they get older, it is harder for them to metabolize alcohol, leading to numerous health risks. It is also important to limit sugars as well as this will greatly benefit the body in other ways such as helping with weight gain. This is because sugar's effect on the body can cause the pancreas to produce less insulin which is crucial for maintaining a healthy lifestyle as an older adult.

Eat Fruits and Vegetables Often

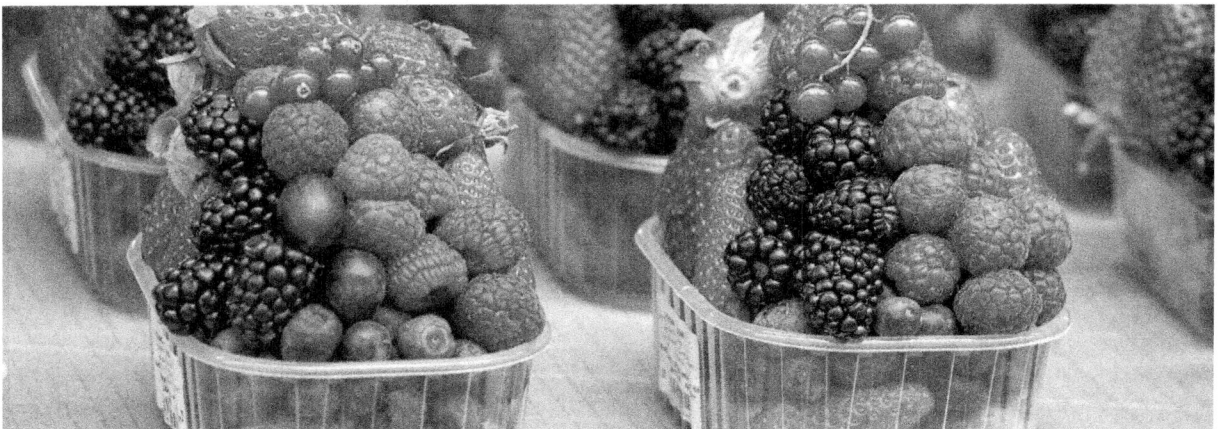

It is important for older adults to eat fruits and vegetables daily. This helps the body stay healthy and gives it the nutrients that it needs to function properly. In addition to this, fruits and vegetables are great for keeping individuals full throughout the day. They also contain lots of fiber which is beneficial for digestion.

Eat at a Set Time Every Day

One of the best ways to ensure eating right is by eating at a set time every day. This way, you will always be sticking to your diet rather than making large changes on different days. Eating at certain times will keep you in check with your body's natural rhythms and help fight off hunger pains.

Eat Enough Fats, Carbohydrates, and Protein

As you get older, your body will not need as much fat. In other words, the less fat you eat, the less fat your body will store. Therefore, it is important for older adults to eat plenty of carbohydrates such as bread, grains, and fruits. Also, you should be eating plenty of protein every day because it is needed for repairing damaged tissues.

Don't Skimp on Water/Juice!

Older adults should drink a gallon or more water per day. This will help increase fluid intake which helps flush out toxins from the body as well as helping keep the kidneys healthy by removing waste products from the body. It is also important to drink plenty of juice, preferably fresh juice from fruits instead of pre-packaged juices.

Avoid Too Much Salt

Many elderlies are on a sodium-restricted diet. This is because it can cause high blood pressure and lead to other complications. It is best to avoid salt as much as possible, especially if you have high blood pressure or heart problems. Instead, try using herbs and spices in your recipes for flavor.

Avoid Getting Too Much Protein and Fat

Because older adults don't metabolize as well as they did when they were younger, eating too much protein and fat can be harmful. It is best to eat healthy sources of protein and fat in moderation such as in fish or lean meats. This is because the protein and fat in most meat are not healthy for older adults.

Enjoy Your Food

If you don't enjoy what you are eating, then why eat it? It doesn't matter if it has fruit or vegetables in it or if it's cooked in a certain way. If you find yourself getting bored or irritated while eating, then take a break and enjoy something else. The point of eating is to enjoy your food so make sure to do this!

Keto Diet for Over 50

A ketogenic diet is a nutritional approach that has been practiced since the 1920s, and it involves eating foods that are very low in carbohydrates and high in fats (the sources of calories). It involves using oils or fats as the primary source of nutrition.

The loss of appetite brought on by the diet may be due to some inherent deficiency, or it can be caused by the removal of certain foods from the diet. "Certain carbohydrate-dense foods like potatoes would appear to be out because they are associated with inflammation," says Dr. Axe. "But if you eat fermented foods—like sauerkraut, kefir, or kombucha—you may find that your symptoms improve. These foods, especially the probiotics in them, may also help restore gut health and improve digestion."

The keto diet has an "immunomodulatory and anti-inflammatory effect" on the body, which means it can be helpful for reducing symptoms of autoimmune conditions.

The ketogenic diet transforms your body into a fat-burning machine. Your muscles break down fat to use as energy instead of carbohydrates (glucose). The liver converts any extra fat into ketones, then sends them to your bloodstream. This is accomplished by severely restricting your carb intake (to about 5% of your total calories) and replacing it with protein plus healthy fats.

There are many benefits to being in ketosis. It helps with many different health conditions—diabetes, epilepsy, cancer, chronic inflammation, Parkinson's, Alzheimer's, and more.

Psychologists say that a high-fat diet can be beneficial for older adults. They point out that people in their 60s and 70s tend to eat less fat than people in their 20s or 30s do. But too much fat can be harmful. It raises cholesterol levels and leads to atherosclerosis or hardening of the arteries. Some research shows that saturated fats increase blood sugar levels and that trans fats lead to greater amounts of belly fat and cardiometabolic disease (heart disease).

Importance of Doctor's Opinion Before Starting the Diet

Your doctor will recommend a balance between fat and carbohydrates. For some older adults with health problems, especially with diabetes, may want you to limit your carb intake and increase the amount of fat in your diet to improve heart health. Recently, we have seen a shift toward the keto diet with many older adults on this type of diet for their cholesterol levels.

Importance of Cholesterol

The "bad cholesterol" in the blood is oxidized low-density lipoprotein or LDL. It leads to plaque deposits on the walls of the arteries and thus narrows down the blood flow. This process is called atherosclerosis.

It is recommended that old adults who are obese try a ketogenic diet. This can reverse many changes in their body such as high cholesterol, high blood pressure, and diabetes. In studies involving older adults, this type of diet has led to dramatic weight loss and improved heart health.

"In a study comparing low versus high-fat diets, researchers found that over a six-year period as many as 14% of women who consumed a low-fat diet died, while only 5% of those on a high-fat diet died," said Dr. Axe.

When older adults have heart disease, it is very beneficial to try the keto diet, especially if they are unable to exercise. This type of diet leads to increased weight loss and is much easier to follow for older adults.

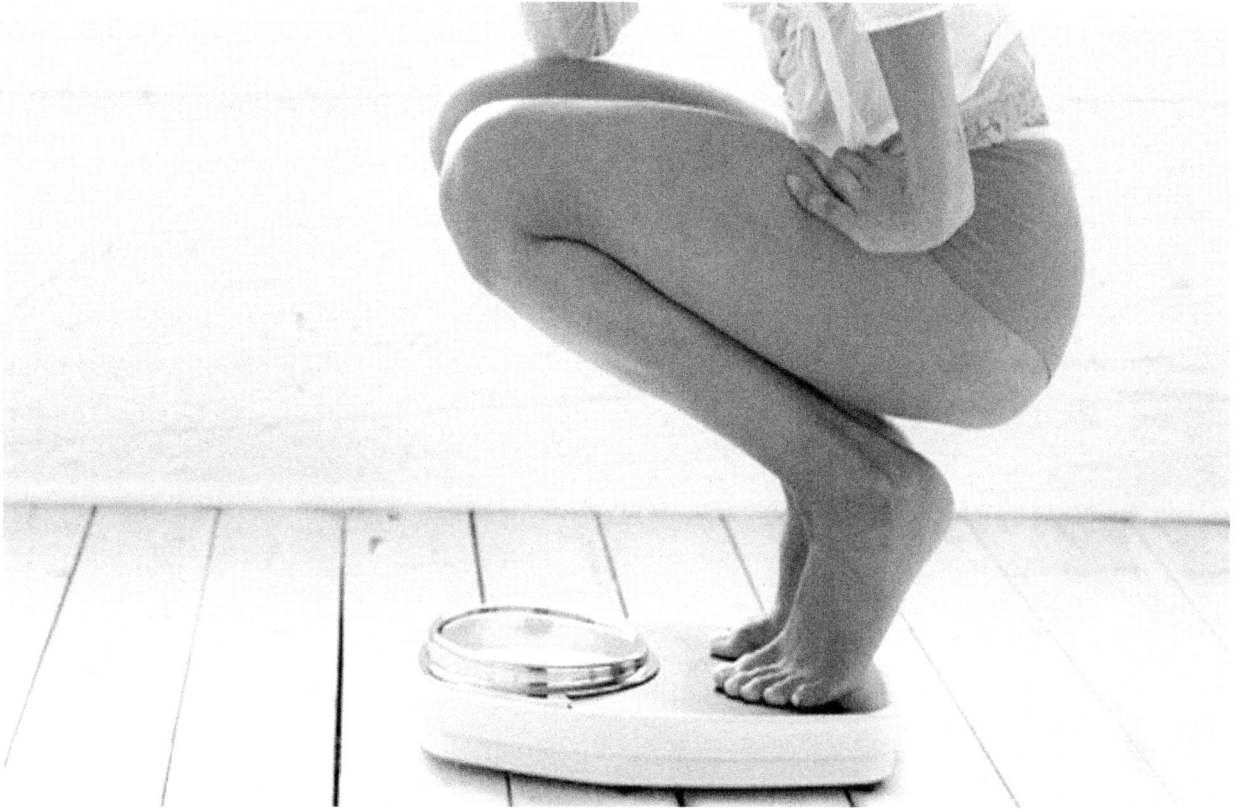

You will need to be more careful of what you eat. Choose foods that are high in fat, but low in carbs. There is less of a chance of gaining weight since the fat slows down the digestive process, and there is less being absorbed into your body (diets with refined carbohydrates which can lead to weight gain). Another benefit is that it will improve cholesterol levels (lower blood pressure and risk of heart disease). If you've tried other diets and had no success, it may be time to try a ketogenic diet.

A keto diet can improve your health by increasing its ability to burn fat and increase its levels of good cholesterol or "good" fats. So, if you want to reduce your weight and improve your health, this is a great way to do it.

One thing that has caused confusion among older adults is the high-fat content. This diet involves eating fats found in olive oil, coconut oil, and meat, instead of carbohydrates found in bread or grain cereals. This can lead to greater calorie intake.

The keto diet is not recommended for people with certain health conditions like diabetes, extreme obesity, or eating disorders (anorexia). Their doctor may recommend a low-calorie diet as an alternative to the ketogenic diet.

Studies show that people who took part in this diet lost more weight than those who didn't consume fats in their diets.

Keto Diet and Aging

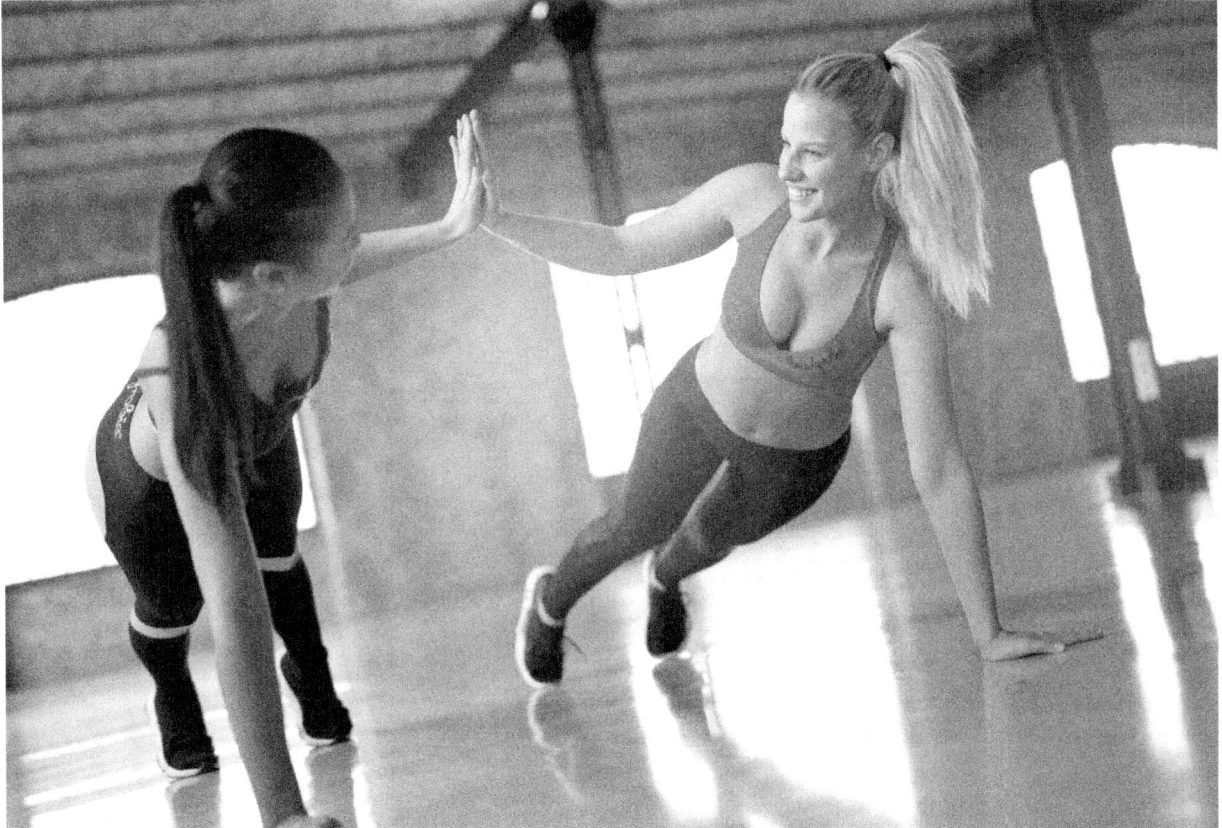

As people get older, they tend to lose muscle mass. Therefore, some people have a difficult time getting started with the diet. Being in ketosis helps you to reduce your overall muscle mass while maintaining a healthy body weight.

You'll learn to eat healthier, and the food will taste so much better! You will experience less pain and tiredness because of increased energy levels from ketosis. In a few short weeks or months, you should notice a difference in your energy levels as well as your mood.

Effects of Ketosis on People Over 50

When you follow a ketogenic diet, your body switches to using fat for fuel rather than the glucose (carbohydrate) your liver and muscles were using before. This process gives you the energy to carry out daily tasks. By eating foods rich in healthy fats, your keto diet gives the body the food it needs for its cells and its organs to function properly.

With a healthy food supply from ketosis, your blood pressure will improve, and you could start reducing your medications or stopping them altogether.

Ketosis helps improve cholesterol levels as well. Because of this, you'll find that even if you have diabetes or high blood pressure, you'll still be able to manage it more easily when on this diet.

The keto diet also gives your body more energy. You'll be able to do the things you want to do several hours longer because of its increased strength. Your body will be able to go a little longer before "burning out," and you'll be able to get on with your life without needing a lot of rest and recovery time.

The keto diet has been shown in recent studies to help with panic disorders, bipolar depression, epilepsy, migraines, and chronic pain. It has the potential to reduce inflammation and reverse many degenerative diseases like Alzheimer's disease.

Intake of Fiber While on Keto Diet for Over 50

When you're on a ketogenic diet, it's best to get about 30 to 40 grams of fiber each day. This is because fiber helps to clear your arteries and keeps your colon healthy.

When you're on a ketogenic diet, you can keep this in check by eating lean protein (about 80 grams of protein each day). Include some healthy fat like avocado or nuts in the process.

You should also avoid sugary foods and drinks. Sugar is known to raise your sugar levels and reduce good cholesterol.

Since the ketogenic diet will make you lose weight, there's a chance your skin could look saggy or wrinkled. If you want to tighten up the skin on your face, neck, or chest, take some coconut oil or massage it directly into your skin at least three times a week. This may improve the appearance of wrinkles around your eyes and mouth when you're in ketosis.

If you're over 50 years old and have high cholesterol, high blood pressure, and type 2 diabetes, try out this new diet plan under the supervision of a doctor.

Regulating Your Hormones with Keto Diet

Hormones regulate the entire process of creating energy in the body. But as we age, our hormone levels start to change to better protect us against illnesses and maintain proper bodily functions.

If you're over 50 years old and your doctor has recommended the keto diet, this diet focuses on low-carb foods that will help with balancing your hormones naturally.

Some women also experience a problem during their menstrual cycle which leads to irregular periods or no period at all. The body uses more calories for the reproductive system when it is in ketosis versus when it is not. Therefore, you may notice you are becoming exhausted after just a few hours of fasting each day on this diet plan.

If you feel like you need to take medications for your cholesterol, blood pressure, or diabetes, talk with your doctor about using the keto diet.

They will be able to help you practice this diet in a controlled manner that will ensure your health doesn't suffer. It's important to work with your doctor because if you have a heart condition or kidney disease, this can cause further deterioration to your health.

The keto diet is shown in studies to enhance fertility for women who are having difficulty conceiving.

What Should You Do While on Keto Diet?

Don't be discouraged if you're 50 or older and go on the ketogenic diet. It's best to consult with your doctor before trying this diet plan, but once you've talked with them and they've supervised you for a few weeks, go ahead and try it!

Not only will the keto diet give you more energy than other diets, but it will also make your body healthier as well.

Remember that even as we age, we can still enjoy life! The keto diet allows us to enjoy tasty foods that are very healthy for us—and for a lifetime.

Is It Safe to Do Keto Diet After 50?

Yes, it's very safe to do a keto diet after 50.

The keto diet after 50 makes you feel good about yourself and gives your body the energy it needs to do all the things you've been wanting to do!

Hormones help regulate how your body reacts to different things. After 50 years old, hormones can be used differently or not at all. As with anything else in life, there are always pros and cons and with this diet, there are some cons that may turn you off.

It is said that for every 100 calories from carbohydrates consumed, the production of insulin will increase by about 30% while fat produces more than double the amount that sugar does. But what happens if you eat 100 calories from fat only? Well, since consuming just one gram of fat has more than twice the number of calories as carbs, that's going to produce a lot more insulin. Insulin is a hormone that is released when you eat carbs and helps your body break them down into glucose, which it uses for energy.

When you're in a state of ketosis, your body can break down fat into fatty acids and use that as energy.

The keto diet also helps with weight loss because you eat fewer calories than before and can spend them on healthier foods. The natural properties found in many foods are good for your health such as calcium and magnesium, but also good for weight loss.

How to Follow Keto Diet Safely?

If you're 50 years or older, it's best to talk with your doctor before trying a ketogenic diet. They will be able to help you use the diet in a controlled manner that will keep your body in balance while safely losing weight.

While many people do the keto diet for weight loss, there are also those that follow the keto diet to help with various medical conditions. It's important to consult with a doctor before trying this diet plan.

The keto diet also helps with fertility in women who are trying to get pregnant. Those that have PCOS (polycystic ovary syndrome), or insulin-resistant diabetes can benefit from this new way of eating.

Be sure you are getting enough calcium, magnesium, and vitamins D and B12 while on this diet plan as part of the healthy lifestyle it promotes. These will help with weight loss, provide for better energy, and regulate your health.

This diet plan is just one of the many types of diets you can try to lose weight and improve your overall health. It's a great idea to consult with a medical professional before changing your diet—especially if you're over 50.

Manage New Habits After 50

As we get older, our minds don't work as fast as they used to. We forget more things than we used to. This is just a part of the aging process and there's not much we can do about it!

Did you know that your brain will continue to lose neurons by the thousands each year? It's true, and since this is happening, we need to change what ways of helping our brain remember things better?

The keto diet encourages memory benefits by offering up new types of food for your body to use for energy. By consuming fat and low carbs, your body goes in a different state where it will begin using these healthy foods instead of continuing to break them down into glucose (sugar).

Try to repeat this process daily, and you'll eventually see the effects of the keto diet on your brain.

The keto diet can also help with sleep by helping your body use the food it eats better. This helps your body relax and rejuvenate so you can get a good night's rest.

You will also be consuming more fat from foods such as meat, fish, and dairy products that will help with weight loss and brain functioning. Many people using this diet plan say it's also an energy booster as well!

Buying organic eggs is another great way to have a healthier lifestyle.

The best part about the keto diet is it's a lifestyle and not just a fad diet. It really helps you change your body—and your mind!

How to Minimize Side Effects of Ketosis

While using the keto diet, there are a few sides affects you need to be aware of.

Too Much Protein Can Lead to Kidney Problems and Other Inflammation

Too much calcium can cause your blood pressure to rise and too much salt will increase your risk for heart-related issues. You want to stay away from these problems as best you can!

Sleeping Issues

Many people find they have trouble sleeping while on this diet plan. This occurs because your body is going through some changes while it adjusts to the new diet. To help with this, you can drink unsweetened tea or water before bed. You can also try taking magnesium supplements if you'd like, but you probably won't need to!

Your body needs more rest as we age, so don't be worried if it takes a little more time to fall asleep at night.

Constipation

The keto diet also causes some issues with your digestive system while it adjusts to the food choices you're making. Upping your water intake along with adding some more fiber to your diet will help things move along a little faster.

All in all, if you want to try the keto diet, it's important to go slowly and make sure you have enough food and water. Many men and women find that this diet plan works for them!

Walk 3-5 times a week or join a gym or join a swimming-pool

The miraculous principles of physical exercises still apply as it always has—just wear your gym shoes and go out for a walk or join a gym and start slowly with cardio exercises or wear a swimming suit and join a pool.

You will notice day by day improvement in your body and mood, you'll discover a difference in how you feel every day. Your energy levels will go up as you are burning fat from your cells and start your body-brain cleaning process.

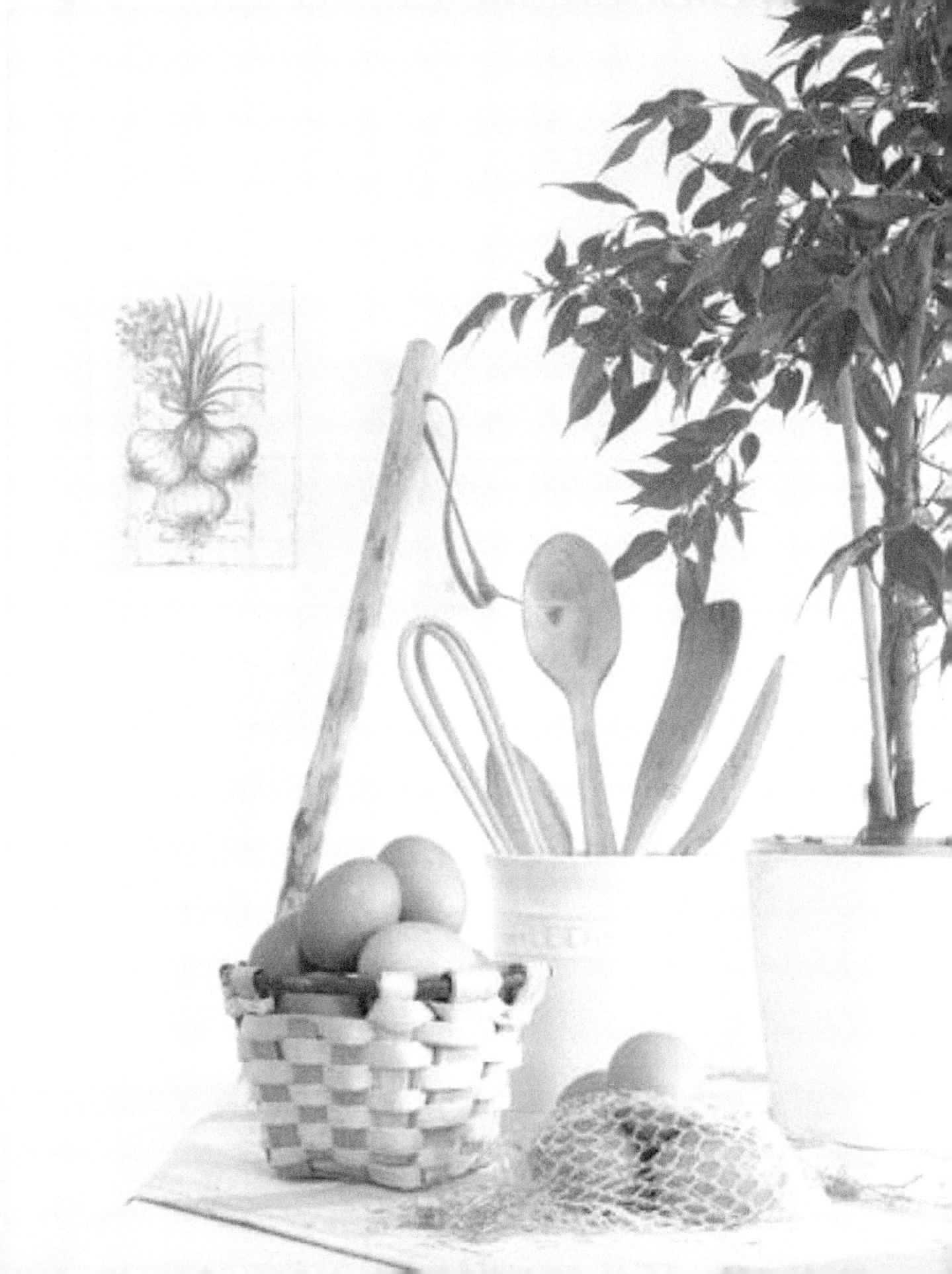

Chapter 3. Kitchen Equipment and Gold Tips

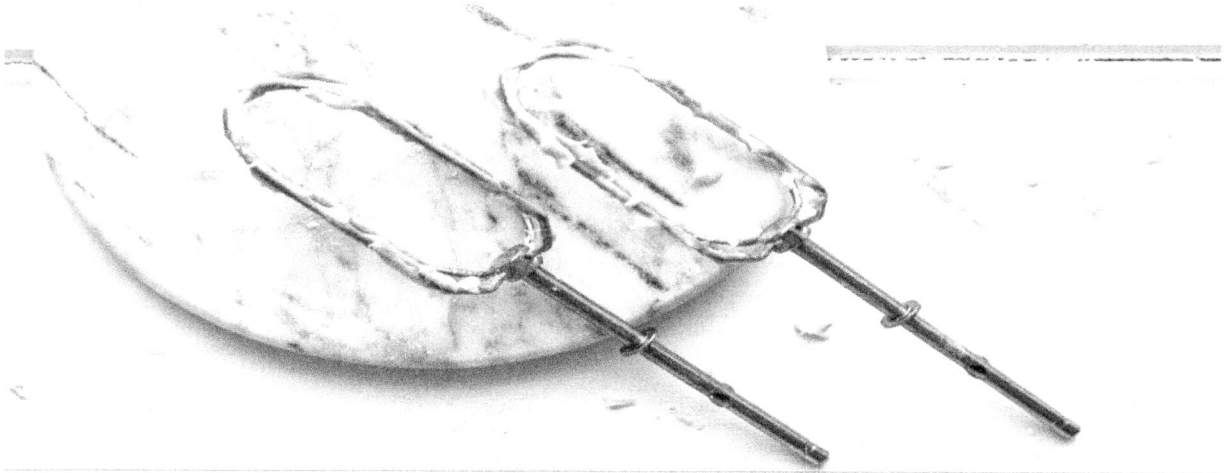

We're going to cover kitchen equipment and gold tips for the ketogenic diet. As a reminder, a ketogenic diet is low in carbs and high in fat content. It's an excellent way to eat if you're looking to lose weight or lower your cholesterol. This is also one of the best diets if you have type 2 diabetes. By cutting carbs from your daily food intake, your body will be sent into ketosis, which burns fat as its primary source of fuel instead of glucose (sugar).

Kitchen Equipment

Here is some kitchen equipment that will help you prepare meals for your keto diet:

1. **Mug:** The best coffee mug for a ketogenic diet is stainless steel. It will keep your coffee warm for hours and help you prepare your healthy meals faster.

2. **Chop-top:** This is the pot that's used to prepare food on the stovetop. The edging helps to keep the contents inside the pot in place, so you don't waste any water, juice, or spices while cooking.

3. **Liquid measuring cup:** If you are buying a liquid measuring cup, choose a glass one over a plastic one as plastic one tends to break easily and may end up leaking your liquid ingredients inside.

4. **Blender:** The best blender for the ketogenic diet is Vitamix. It can grind almost everything you throw at it, including nuts, seeds, and even coffee beans!

5. **Cutting board:** The best cutting board is bamboo or wood. Avoid using plastic ones if possible because it has been found that they are hard to sanitize and may contain toxic chemicals like BPA and Phthalates which are harmful to your health.

6. **Saucepan:** Choose a saucepan with a capacity of 3–4 quarts, the bigger the better as it will save you time when cooking for the whole family.

7. **Mixer:** The one you choose will depend on the food you wish to mix. If you are preparing salad dressing or whisking eggs, go for a traditional hand mixer or immersion blender because they can do the job without the fuss of a regular mixer.

8. **Grater:** The bag grater is great if you are looking for a quick way to get some shredded veggies or cheese into your salad dressings. But if you're using it in the kitchen, safety is of utmost concern, so make sure it's conical, has stainless steel blades, and that it's dishwasher safe.

9. **Cutting knife:** A good quality knife is essential for any kitchen, especially if you're making many salads and green vegetables. You'll need to use it to chop all your ingredients.

10. **Whisk:** Egg whiskers are usually made for mixing the egg yolk and incorporate air into the eggs when making, e.g., Hollandaise sauce or meringue. But they can also be used to mix ingredients in a blender or food processor, like flour, if you are about to make pancakes or bread!

11. **Vegetable peeler:** The best vegetable peeler is one that has a sharp blade and doesn't take off too much of the vegetable as you are peeling it. It's perfect to have

one that removes thin strips that you can use to wrap around the meat to make a nice-looking appetizer.

12. **Meat pounder:** If you're preparing meat for some dishes, it's good to have a meat pounder in your kitchen as it will save you time and energy rather than using your fist or any other utensils around.

13. **Milk frothier:** This is perfect for making a hot or cold mocha latte with your favorite coffee. It can also be used in making thin milkshakes such as a sugar-free strawberry milkshake recipe.

14. **Pastry brush:** This flat brush is ideal for brushing egg whitewash or olive oil onto a dish or pan to give it that lovely shiny finish it requires before cooking.

15. **Cake tester:** If you're baking some cakes, pies, or muffins, it's a must-have kitchen tool that will ensure you have that perfect consistency of the batter and baked product.

16. **Grater with a pouring bag:** This is ideal for grating, pressing, or crushing your zest or citrus fruits into your favorite recipes.

17. **Kitchen scale:** A kitchen scale is an indispensable tool in any kitchen. It allows you to keep track of the amount of food you put in the fridge and helps you with portion control. For instance, if you buy 3 kg of avocados for your next recipe, measure them all out before entering the fridge so that when it's time for that recipe again, you will know exactly how many avocados are left to use!

18. **Corkscrew:** If you like drinking wine, this is the one kitchen utensil that will not only save you a lot of time but also make it easy for you to open those pesky wine bottles.

19. **Julienne peeler:** This is like a regular vegetable peeler, but instead of thin strips, it produces small thin sticks that are perfect for making your own stir fry or salad.

20. **Potato ricer:** If you come across the term "mashed potatoes" on the ketogenic diet, then this is what you'll need! It's a tool for pressing the moisture out of potatoes so they become nice and fluffy.

21. **Scale, salter, or refrigerator:** If you plan to measure or weigh food in the portioned containers, you will need a scale and if it's not digital, then make sure it has a reasonable LCD display with an easy-to-use knob.

22. **Cookie sheets:** The best cookie sheet is one that has easily removable non-stick coating, so your cookies don't stick to it while they are in the oven or once you put them on your plate.

23. **Spatula:** A silicone spatula is ideal for spreading and scraping. It's a good addition to have one of these because you can use it on the stovetop too, rather than just on the baking dish when you are cooking.

24. **Flat measuring cups:** If you like to bake cookies or bread, it's important to measure your ingredients accurately and measure them in the right portions to keep track of how full each container is. It's also important to have accurate measurements so that you don't end up using too much of an ingredient, thus affecting the flavor of your product!

Recommended Foods

When getting started with your keto diet, I suggest you consume the following foods:

- **Healthy fats:** Focus on adding in as much fat as possible and eliminate processed and saturated fat. It's not essential that you consume a lot of animal products as a keto dieter. You can start with consuming some eggs and salmon to get your omega 3s easily from food.

- **Fiber sources:** Add fiber to your diet by eating plenty of green veggies like broccoli, kale, and spinach. These foods act as a great source of fiber and will help to keep your body full.

- **Carbohydrates:** Add starch to your diet by eating vegetables such as cauliflower, zucchini, and asparagus.

- **Fat sources:** You can consume the following forms of fat on the ketogenic diet:
  - ➢ Avocados are a great way to get healthy fats easily. They are also super tasty when eaten alone or with some salt and lemon juice.
  - ➢ Olives can be consumed in small amounts, but they should not be eaten too often because of the high amount of salt they contain.
  - ➢ Olive oil is high in fat as well and it's a healthier option than butter.

- **Coconut oil:** Most people have heard of coconut oil by now because of the various health benefits it portrays. You can use coconut oil as a butter substitute, a massage/facial moisturizer, or a hair glossier! There are many other ways you

- can use it so be creative and start experimenting!

Gold Tips for Ketogenic Diet

- **Eating out should be avoided:** This is something I feel very adamant about because when you're eating out, you are not in control of what you're ingesting. Some restaurants like to add unhealthy saturated fats and sugars into their dishes. If you have no choice, then do your research online and try to find the restaurant that has the lowest amount of fat and sugar in their meals.

- **Carry snacks:** When traveling or visiting someone who is not keto-friendly, it's good to have some snacks in your bag so that you can still stick to your diet with ease.

- **Drink plenty of water:** This is very important and something that's often forgotten. The ketogenic diet tends to dehydrate you. Make sure you drink at least 2 liters a day and add lots of ice to your drinks, so you get more water into your system.

- **Eat whole foods:** When possible, choose whole foods over processed foods. Whole foods contain less sugar and fat, so they are better for the ketogenic diet.

- **Empty out your kitchen:** If you have tons of unhealthy junk food in your home, it will be very easy to simply grab some snacks or meals when you're hungry and it will probably be easier to give up on the diet this way. Try to keep your kitchen clear of excess food so that it's easier to stick to the diet.

- **Do not go back on the diet:** I know that this is something you want, but don't give in just yet. The last time we lost weight, it was easy to start the diet and we didn't have as many cravings when we were eating healthy. However, after a certain point, our bodies started adapting and it became harder for us to stay on our diet. If you've been keto before then I suggest waiting until you reach your goal or pre-set weight goal before going back on the diet. Reduce your calories slightly and start with a low-carb day to see how you feel. If you don't like it, then you are free to go back on the diet.

- **Keep a food journal:** This is especially true if you're not very familiar with what foods contain what nutrients. It's important to keep track of your portion sizes and the calories that you consume each day so that you don't end up eating more than your daily calorie limit.

- **Include physical activity in your routine:** This is important because being on a diet and not moving much can cause you to gain weight. Your body needs exercise so it can burn up fat and keep your metabolism going strong.

These are things that I changed in my lifestyle with regards to the ketogenic diet and how I started to feel healthier.

- **I started drinking 8 glasses of water a day:** Drinking water is so important because it helps you to hydrate your body and keeps your body running as smoothly as possible. Many people forget about this aspect of their diet, but the results are astounding, it's easier to stay active without feeling hungry all the time.

- **I started doing yoga:** Many people do yoga at home, but I suggest that you join a local class. Not only will it help you stay active, but you'll also learn some great poses that can be incorporated into pranayama exercises, which are essential for staying healthy on the ketogenic diet.

- **I started sleeping more:** This is so important because sleep will help to lower your cravings. People tend to eat things when they're feeling tired or lazy. Make sure you get a good night's rest because this will help to keep your binge-craving in check.

- **I started taking cold shower:** This is revitalizing for body and brain, releases endorphins, and you have an absolutely great feeling to face your daily routine more energized and focused.

- **I started taking hot baths:** Hot baths are great for burning off excess water in your body and keeping yourself warm during the colder months. They also help to relax muscles and help to relieve pain from soreness or injuries. Baths can be very therapeutic so make sure you try to schedule one every week.

- **I started using yoga-meditation:** I found that meditation helps me feel more relaxed during my day, just start with 10 minutes of long breath and relaxing in butterfly yoga pose (standard pose sitting with your hands clasped on feet, straight back, heels close to pelvis, bring outer knees down, soles together edge of feet on the floor). It's great for your body and mind so make sure you give it a try!

- **I started keeping to myself**: This might be hard because family is important but if you don't want them to know that you're on a diet (which they shouldn't know in the first place) then just keep them out of it. Your body is not theirs and they should not have any say in what you eat or lose.

- **I started drinking my coffee black:** This is something big that many people do not realize. All the caffeine that you consume goes directly to your liver so when you drink black coffee, you are not taking in so much of the harmful effects of caffeine. You still get your fix of energy and focus from a cup of coffee, but all those unwanted calories are burned off with the caffeine.

- **I started eating more vegetables**: I know that this might sound absurd because everyone loves meat, but certain vegetables have very little fat or calories and can be very filling without feeling full. I still make sure to include plenty of meat in my meals, but I take an extra serving of vegetables and mix it into my meals. I also make sure to keep an eye out for the fat and calorie counts on my items so that I can buy the most nutritious ones to help me stay on track.

- **I started taking multivitamins:** I like selecting vitamins that are good for my body and easy for me to fit into my daily routine. My favorite multivitamin is one from Thorne Research, where they have everything, you could ever want in a vitamin supplement at a great price with no additives or fillers.

- **I started exercising more:** I know that this might not be something you expect to have on your "lifestyle changes" list, but exercising is very important. I suggest that you try to get outside and walk or run every day. Even if it's only five minutes of your day, make sure that you get yourself moving because exercise is the best way to keep your body shape and burn fat.

- **Don't be afraid to get extra help:** If you need extra help with your diet, don't be afraid to seek advice from friends or experts in the field. If you can't get started on a certain diet for whatever reason, then give another one a try. So many diets change over time so you never know what the best one for you will be.

Ketosis is an amazing way to lose weight and improve your overall health, but it will not work for everyone. I like the keto diet because it has been very successful for me, however, it's important that you do your research and understand things such as whether your body can adapt to a high-fat diet. That's why I suggest trying out different ketogenic diets before settling on one that looks appealing to you.

Chapter 4. Keto Join Med Diet

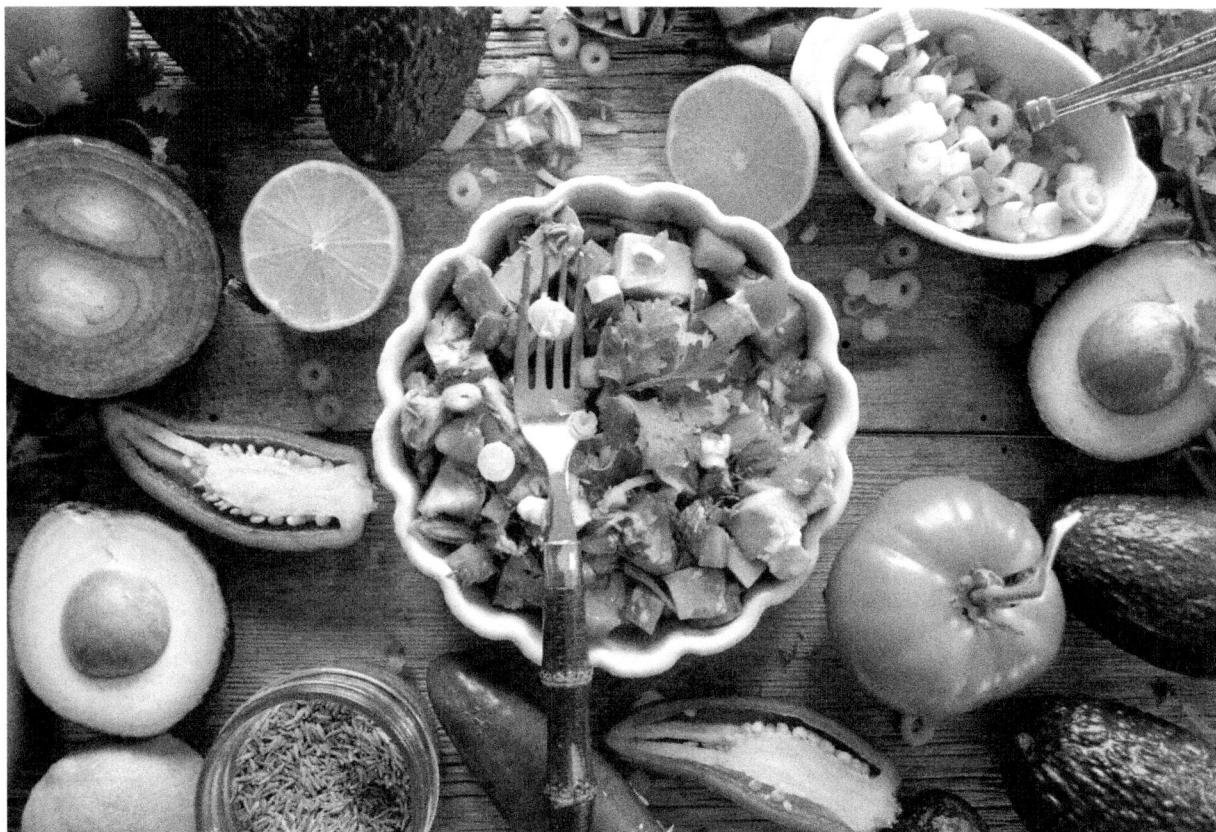

What Is Mediterranean Diet?

Mediterranean diet is a **"way of life"** is also a group of related foods originating in the cuisine of countries bordering the Mediterranean Sea. It is associated with the countries in Southern Europe, Greece, Italy, and Spain. The diet shares common characteristics with other healthy diets, but it includes significant amounts of strategic nutrients not eaten in other diets, such as blue fresh fish, fresh vegetables, and fresh fruits, nuts, and legumes, strictly avoiding processed and industrial foods.

The Mediterranean diet has been found to be one that help lower risk factors for cardiovascular disease without medications or surgery. In fact, about 80% of people on these diets will live longer than those who do not follow this lifestyle model. Some of the Mediterranean diet methods include usually eating foods that are naturally low in saturated fats, high in monounsaturated fats, or polyunsaturated fats. For example, olives are used in making pasta and sauces as well as grilled meats. In addition, nuts are also eaten regularly on this diet, including nut butter made with olive oil along with almonds and peanuts.

Does the Mediterranean Diet Cause Weight Loss?

There is no black or white answer to this—it's just a matter of what you consider following diet advice. If weight loss is defined as losing more than 5 pounds per week, with the help of daily body exercises, is evident that you cannot achieve your goal without training. The high fiber intake and low-calorie nature of this diet, only, don't make it conducive for weight loss. The concern with this diet when it comes to weight loss is that individuals are unable to sacrifice themselves with **daily training**. Exercise our body and brain every day is the real **miracle** that can drive us to lose weight. Increase the awareness of the daily training benefits is extremely useful to help our brain to gain general wellness. It is so challenging how all the vital Live's things. Changing bad habits is the **first step**, to manage. To be sure to achieve positive results in the long-term base, daily physical activity and new healthy lifestyle habits for **weighting loss** are a "Must"

Similarities of Ketogenic and Mediterranean Diet

In terms of general nutrition, the Mediterranean diet shares many similarities with a ketogenic diet. Both diets are high in fiber, fruits, vegetables, and healthy fats avoiding processed foods.

The ketogenic diet and the Mediterranean diet are also very flexible in food choices and requires no calorie tracking or other such tasks.

In terms of specific health benefits, both Mediterranean and Keto diet has been shown to help reduce factors associated with many common age diseases. These include obesity-related cholesterol levels and hypertension as well as blood pressure when consumed over a long period of time.

Differences of Ketogenic and Mediterranean Diet

The Mediterranean diet is a far cry from the strict nature of the ketogenic diet. This diet is very flexible, requiring no calorie tracking or other restrictions on food intake. It's not as restrictive with daily macronutrient ratios either and encourages daily consumption of carbohydrates and healthy fats. The ketogenic diet on the other hand is restrictive and very difficult. It requires an 80:20 ratio of fat: protein and a strict no-carb count throughout the day. Also, it's unlikely that any high fiber intake would be possible with this level of restriction.

The lack of cereal grains in the Mediterranean diet also makes it incompatible with some ketogenic ideas such as eating only fat or using oils that have been extracted from grain products (such as coconut oil). This could potentially lead to digestive issues, as Greek yogurt would not be tolerated for example. Also, nuts are allowed in the Mediterranean diet, but peanuts are not.

How Compatible Is the Med Diet with a Keto Lifestyle?

The primary issue people encounter when considering whether they can follow this lifestyle model while on a ketogenic diet is carbohydrates. Even though this diet does not restrict total carbohydrate intake, it does require that most of your carbohydrates coming from fiber-rich vegetables and fruits (rather than grains). It's not completely clear why this is important, but there are several theories on the subject.

One of the concerns associated with a ketogenic diet is that it's very difficult to get enough fiber in your diet. The high restrictions on grains could potentially prevent you from getting enough fiber in your diet, which is essential for a healthy digestive system and overall health. In addition, it may also lead to constipation due to the lack of fiber intake on this diet. In general, though, there doesn't appear to be any evidence that shows that a Mediterranean diet needs more fiber than most other diets.

In addition, the high fiber intake of the Mediterranean diet may lead to increased chances of cardiovascular disease. Certainly, it's not advisable to follow this diet if you have pre-existing heart issues.

In general, there is no doubt that this is a healthy dietary pattern, and it also shares some dietary similarities with a ketogenic diet. However, there are major differences between these two types of eating regimens. It's important to keep these differences in mind when considering following a ketogenic diet on top of a Mediterranean style eating method.

Keto Mediterranean Diet

The keto Mediterranean diet is a combination of the Mediterranean Diet and a ketogenic diet. It's very similar to the Mediterranean diet in terms of general nutrition. However, it also allows for small amounts of carbohydrates throughout the day. This is like a ketogenic diet general, but with a higher ratio of fat (75–80% vs. 25–30% on a standard ketogenic diet).

In terms of specific health benefits, the keto Mediterranean diet is milder than a traditional ketogenic diet and is more acceptable for individuals who may be sensitive to transforming their bodies from a carbohydrate burner to an energy powerhouse. Another potential benefit is that this eating scheme could be viewed as sustainable over time, which would reduce potential drawbacks such as intestinal discomfort.

Much of the same issues mentioned above for the Mediterranean diet also apply to the keto Mediterranean diet. There is a very high amount of dietary fiber in both, which could lead to potential problems for individuals with gastrointestinal issues or those who are sensitive to fiber intake. In addition, there's a potential increase in cardiovascular disease risk for those prone to such health concerns. One of the main benefits of a keto diet is that it lowers heart disease risk considerably, however, this benefit may be limited for those with existing conditions who follow this eating plan as well.

Finally, there's also no clear scientific evidence that shows why a high fiber intake is essential for good health when following a ketogenic diet.

Overall, the keto Mediterranean diet is a viable option for those who want to follow a healthier lifestyle and are slightly more willing to closely inspect their diet. While following this diet may be possible, it's important to take the proper precautions and steps to consider how they impact other aspects of your health. A few of these tips include:

Keep in mind that if you eat grains (even if they're technically keto-friendly), you might not be able to adhere to this eating plan due to its regularity in your diet. As mentioned above, try having some nut flours for whenever you feel that you're getting constipated.

If you want to add some plant-based dairy products into your daily routine, try using a full-fat Greek yogurt that's not sweetened. These will likely be more tolerated with the low carb intake required by this diet.

In general, it's best that you remain as active as possible while following this type of diet. Getting the required amount of exercise will not only keep your body and mind healthy, but it will also help you stay more satisfied with your food choices.

It's worth noting that there are studies that show a higher risk of cancer with those who follow vegetarian diets high in carbohydrates. These studies note that people who follow these types of diets have a lower intake of meat and higher intakes of fruits and vegetables. The types of foods or food groups (e.g., high-fiber fruits vs. meats) are often not specified in these studies, so it's difficult to draw any conclusions regarding why these differences occurred. It's also possible that the individuals who ate the vegetarian diet with higher amounts of fruit and vegetables had a lower cancer risk.

While there are clear advantages to following a ketogenic diet (versus a traditional Mediterranean diet), there are also some potential disadvantages. Understanding why these differences occur may help you make an informed decision, however, it's important to remember that while following this eating plan, you will need to learn how to properly adapt your cooking skills or take advantage of pre-made meal alternatives if you choose not to eat certain ingredients or food groups (e.g., full-fat Greek yogurt). Other than that, there are no major changes in your daily routine and eating habits, except that you need to be a bit more vigilant about making sure you're getting enough fat into your diet.

For those who wish to try a keto Mediterranean diet, it's important to remember that this is not the only type of low carb eating plan that is out there. You have plenty of options if you're interested in trying this type of diet for yourself.

Benefits of Keto Mediterranean Diet

There are many reasons why it may be worthwhile to consider following a ketogenic eating plan such as the keto Mediterranean diet. If you're interested in trying it for yourself, here's a quick look at some of the potential benefits that can be found from these types of dietary approaches:

- Many people who follow the ketogenic diet or keto Mediterranean diet find that they have more energy and feel less hungry than they did when following other low carb eating plans.
- Perhaps best of all, following a ketogenic diet has been shown to help you shed body fat, even if you're already at a weight that you consider "fat accepting" (e.g., in the healthy range). Other diets have been shown to help with weight loss but not so much with fat reduction, which is often one of the main goals of a keto plan

as your body will burn much more fat in comparison to carbs when following this type of eating plan.

- In addition, this eating plan can help you lower your glycemic index (how quickly food is digested and released into the bloodstream) which may help reduce the risk of heart disease and diabetes. In general, a keto Mediterranean diet is likely to be better for cardiovascular health than a traditional Mediterranean diet, especially when it comes to maintaining good cholesterol levels.

- A keto Mediterranean diet isn't just for losing weight or improving cardiovascular health; it also has several other potential benefits, including reducing inflammation, fighting off cancer cells in some cases, and helping to maintain a healthy brain.

- It's worth noting that although the keto Mediterranean diet was created by a group of chefs and nutritionists at a culinary institute in Italy, it's not just for those who want to follow a healthy eating plan or lose weight.

- Finally, a keto Mediterranean diet can help improve your memory by reducing inflammation in your brain. This isn't something that's been well established yet, but it's worth noting that there are studies out there showing that high-fat diets may help with brain health

Weight Loss with Keto Mediterranean Diet

If you're looking for a way to lose weight, then a keto Mediterranean diet may be what you're looking for. The good news is that studies involving people following this type of eating plan and **daily training** have shown that you can lose significant amounts of body fat while keeping your blood sugar levels controlled.

Take heart, though: it's not just the fact that you burn more fat than carbs when following a keto Mediterranean diet doing physical exercises every day. You can simply change your mind set about how you look at training. There's also no denying that following this type of fitness plan help to increase your overall intake of self-confidence that is the best fuel for **brainstorming** necessary to switch from bad habits, in better healthy habits.

In general, studies show that a keto Mediterranean diet can help you lose more weight than a traditional eating-training plan. In fact, people following this type of eating-training plan lost an average of 3.3 kg (7.2 pounds) per week, which was significantly more weight than those who don't follow the keto Mediterranean eating-training plan.

You may also want to consider the fact that a keto Mediterranean plan is more likely to keep your weight loss efforts sustainable over the long term. The type of fat you eat also plays a role in whether you'll be able to stick with this eating plan for a long period of time. Keep in mind that a keto Mediterranean diet can lead to faster initial weight loss, associated with training plan, but the matter is to resist to follow the rules at least 8-12 weeks to maintain weight loss long term time.

The consensus on this type of diet seems to be that it works best for people who want to lose weight, and they are sure to change habits and start to do physical exercises every day. If you're looking for a train-fix weight loss plan though, then the keto Mediterranean diet may be something you want to consider.

While there are many challenges with following this type of diet, including issues related to how it fits into your lifestyle, most users report feeling satisfied and more energized when they begin to train every day and see their wellness take place.

In terms of the potential health benefits that can occur when following an eating-training plan like **Keto Med Diet**, most users report relief from their chronic pain while losing weight and seeing their body-brain energy levels improve greatly with daily exercises.

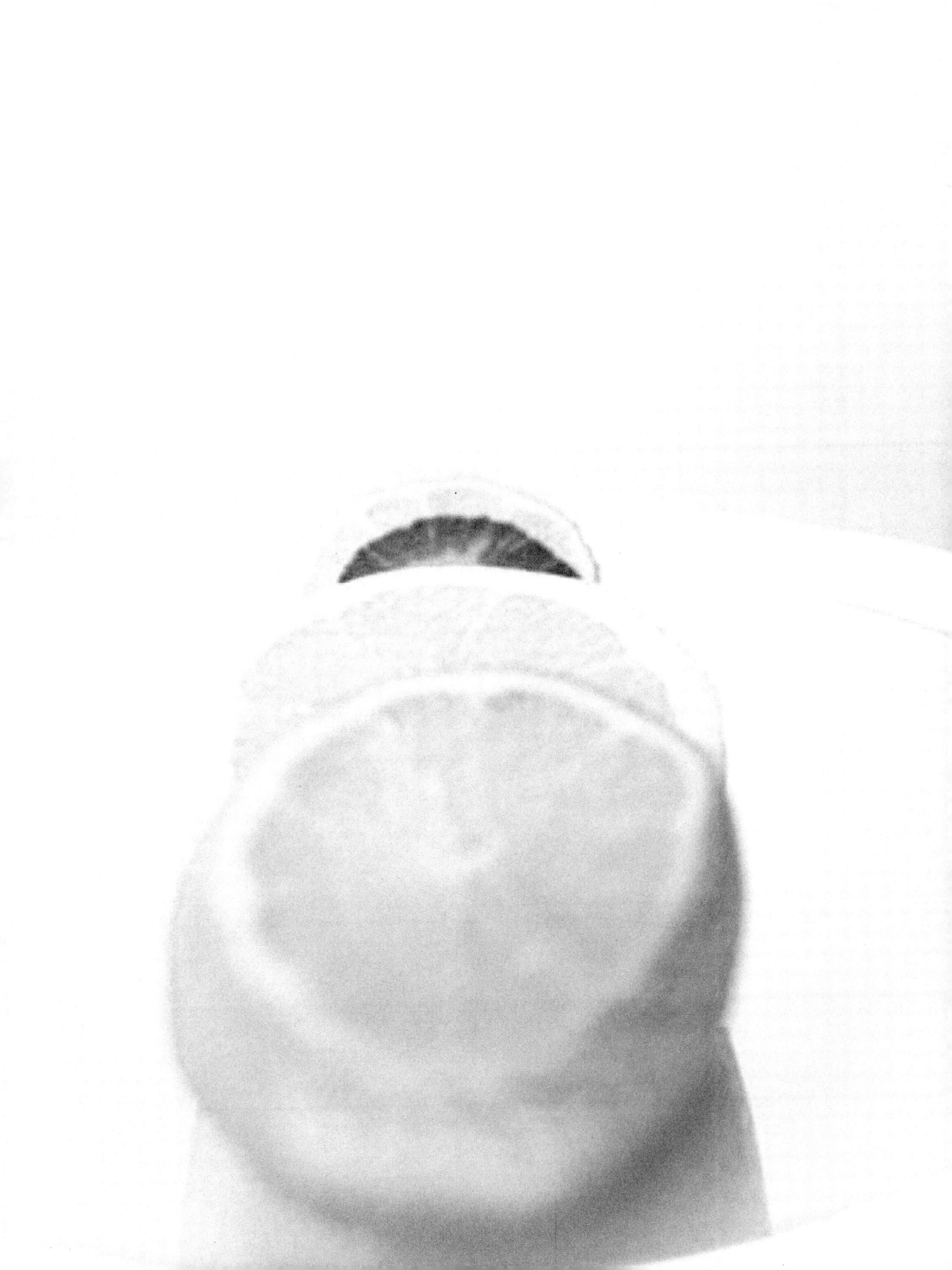

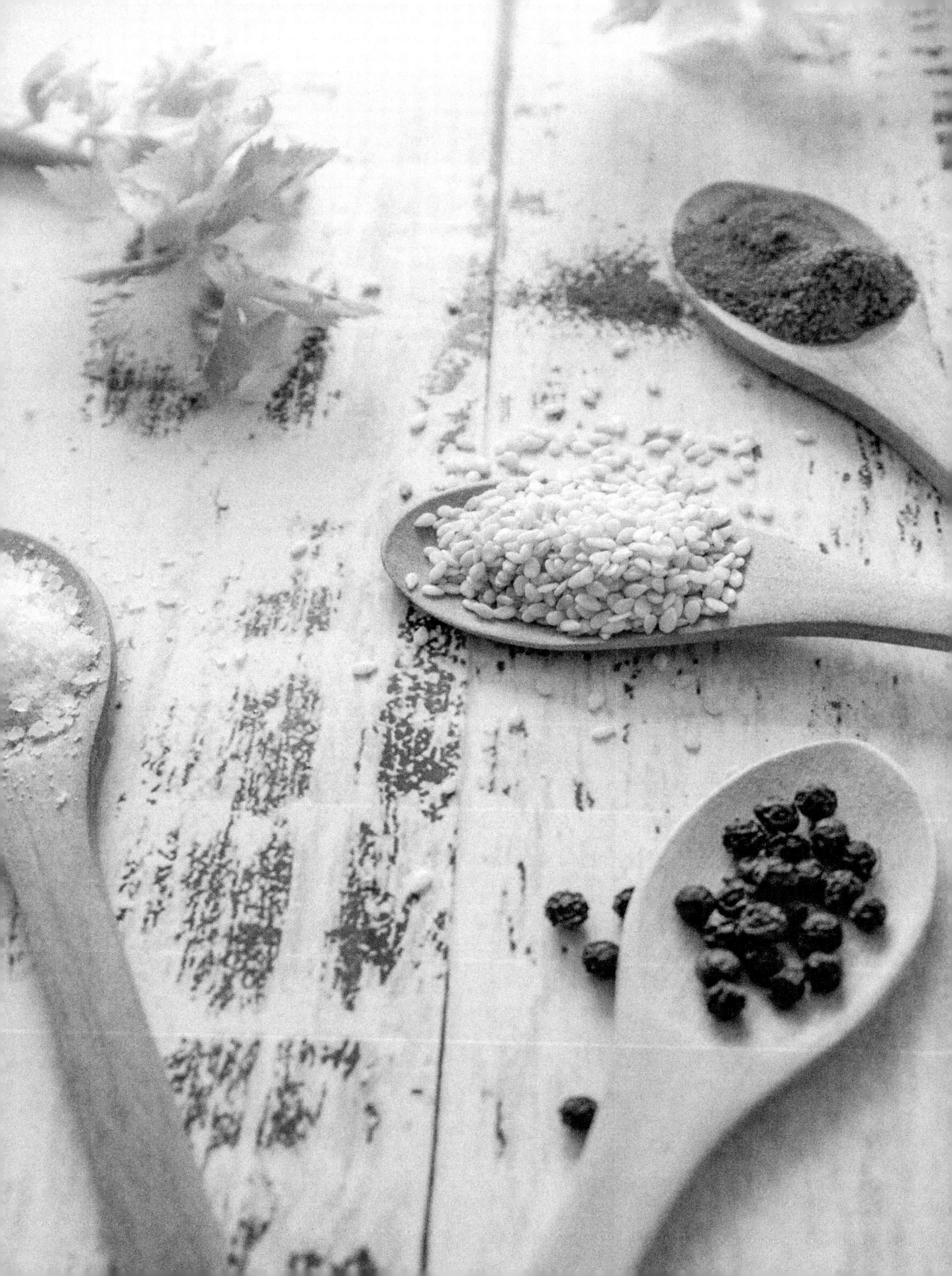

breakfast

snacks

lunch

dinner

veggies

dips

sweets

fruits

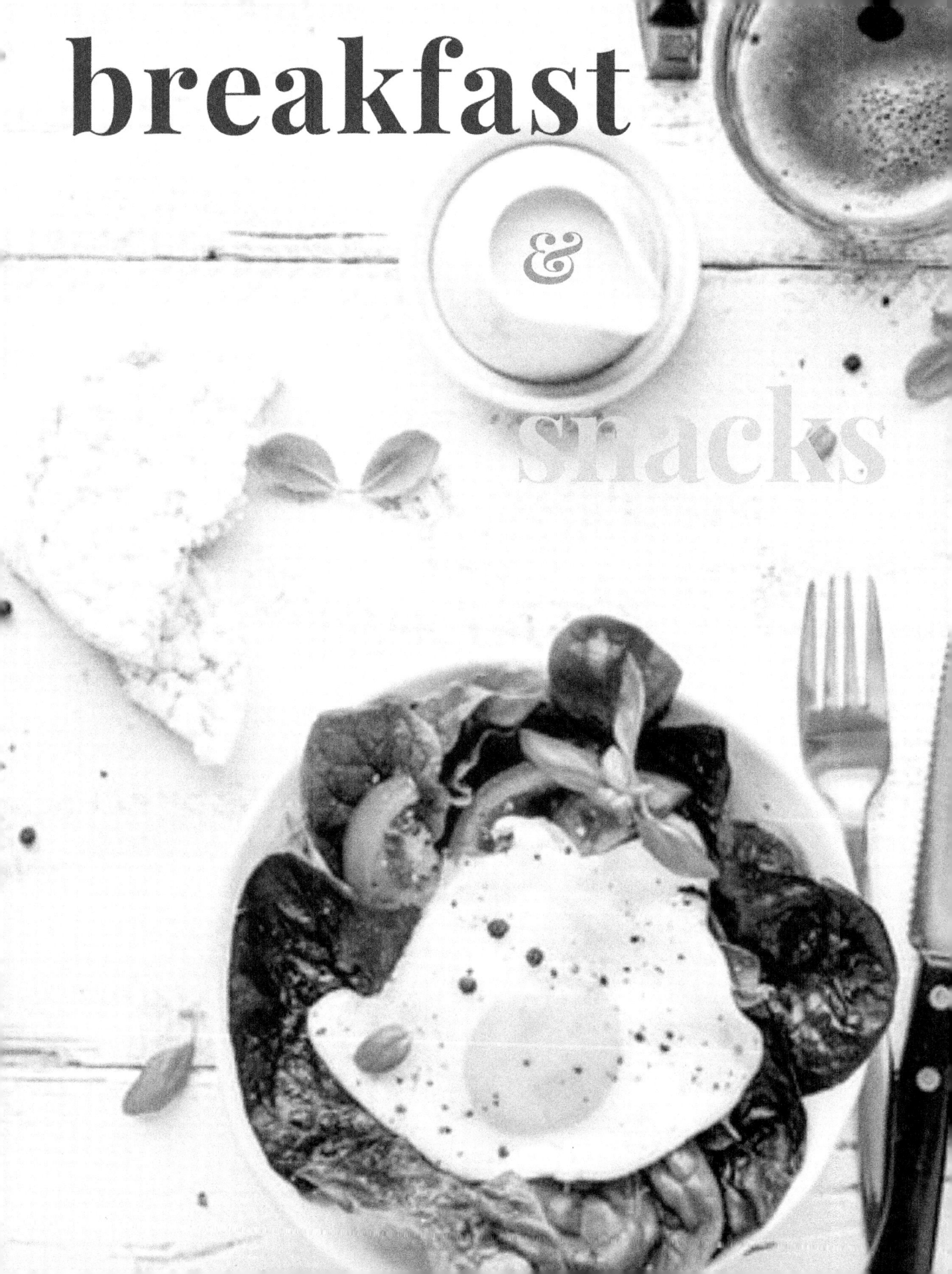

breakfast

&

snacks

1. Bacon and Avocado Omelet

Preparation time: 5 minutes

Cooking time: 5 minutes

Servings: 1

Ingredients:

- 1 slice of crispy bacon
- 2 organic eggs
- 1/2 cup grated parmesan cheese
- 2 tbsp. Ghee
- 1 avocado

Nutrition:

- Calories: 719
- Carbohydrate: 3.3 g
- Fat: 63 g
- Protein: 30 g

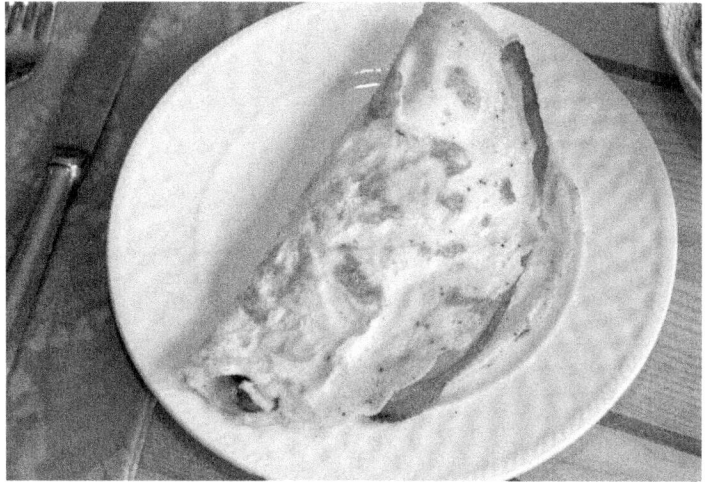

Directions:

1. Cook the bacon and set it aside.
2. Mix the eggs and parmesan cheese.
3. Heat a skillet and add the ghee to melt. Mix in the eggs, then cooks for 30 seconds.
4. Flip and cook again for 30 seconds.
5. Serve with the crunched bacon bits and sliced avocado.

Preparation time: 10 mins

Cooking time: 5 minutes

Servings: 2

Ingredients:

- 1/2 avocado
- 1 tsp. lemon juice
- 2 tsp. capers
- 1 tsp. chopped cilantro
- A pinch crushed red pepper flake
- 2 slices of smoked salmon
- Olive oil to taste
- Salt to taste

Nutrition:

- Calories: 212
- Fat: 11 g
- Carbohydrates: 10 g
- Fiber: 5 g
- Sugar: 2 g
- Protein: 15.6 g

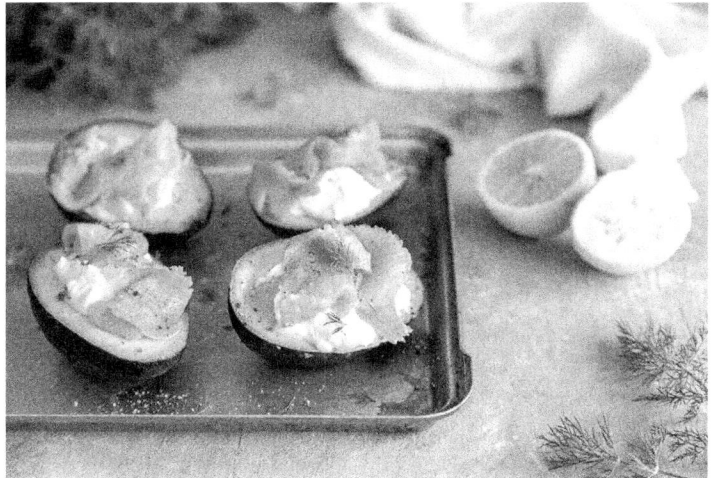

Directions:

1. Scoop the avocado from its skin and place it in a bowl. Add the lemon juice, capers, cilantro, red pepper flakes, olive oil, and salt, and mix well. Slice the salmon into two long strips. Place one of them on each plate. Divide the avocado mixture between the plates or serve on top.

Preparation time: 5 minutes

Cooking time: 2 minutes

Servings: 2

Ingredients:

- 1/3 cup old-fashioned oatmeal
- 1/2 cup unsweetened vanilla almond milk
- 2 tbsp. chopped walnuts
- **Suggested additions:** Vanilla extract, cinnamon, or any other flavorings of choice

Directions:

1. Using your hands, mix the oatmeal with the almond milk and walnuts.
2. Form into a bowl and serve with your favorite toppings, such as additional nuts, strawberries, or blueberries.

Nutrition:

- Calories: 38
- Fat: 1 g
- Carbohydrates: 2 g
- Fiber: 1 g
- Sugar: 0 g
- Protein: 3 g

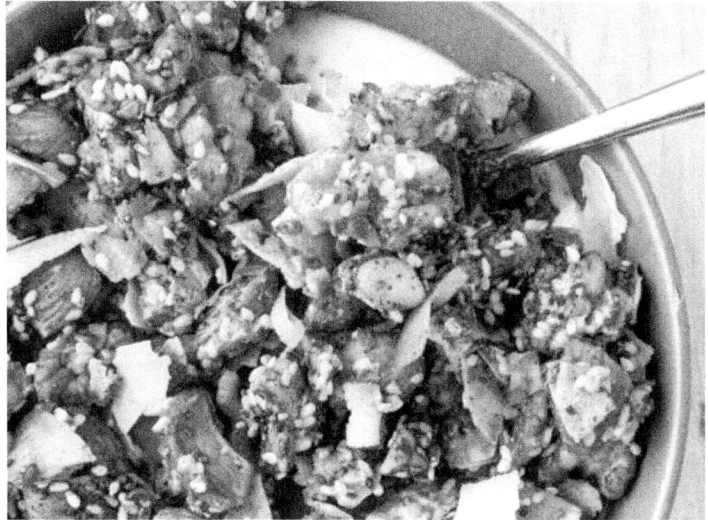

Preparation time: 5 minutes

Cooking time: 4 minutes

Servings: 6

Ingredients:

- 7 oz. kale, chopped (tiny pieces)
- 10 oz. zucchini, washed and grated
- 1 tsp. basil
- 1/2 tsp. salt
- 1/4 cup almond flour
- 1/2 tbsp. mustard
- 1 large egg
- 1 tbsp. coconut milk
- 1 white onion, diced
- 1 tbsp. olive oil

Nutrition:

- Calories: 110
- Carbohydrates: 4 g
- Fat: 5 g
- Protein: 16 g

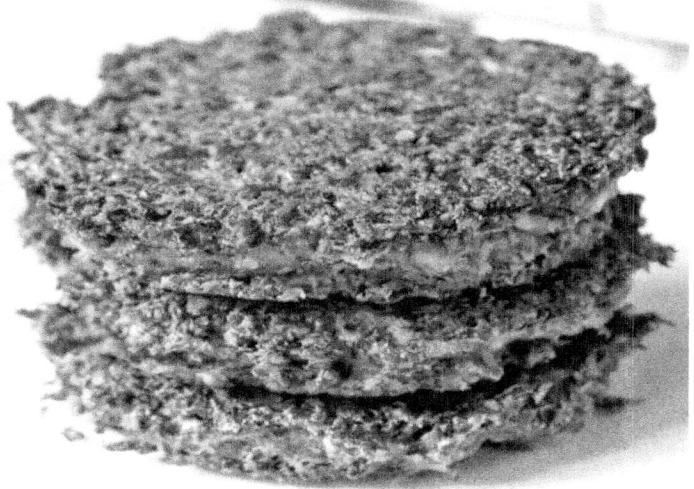

Directions:

1. In a medium bowl, mix kale and zucchini. Add basil and salt and stir. Add almond flour and mustard. Stir well.

2. In another bowl, whisk together egg, coconut milk, and onion. Pour egg mixture into zucchini mixture and knead the thick dough.

3. Preheat the pan with olive oil on medium heat. Shape fritters with the help of a spoon and put them in the pan. Cook fritters for about 2 minutes per side. Transfer fritters to a paper towel to remove excess oil. Serve hot.

Preparation time: 5 minutes

Cooking time: 5 minutes

Servings: 1

Ingredients:

- 1 tbsp. butter
- 2 eggs
- 2 tbsp. soft cream cheese with chives

Nutrition:

- Calories: 341
- Carbohydrates: 3 g
- Fat: 31 g
- Protein: 15 g

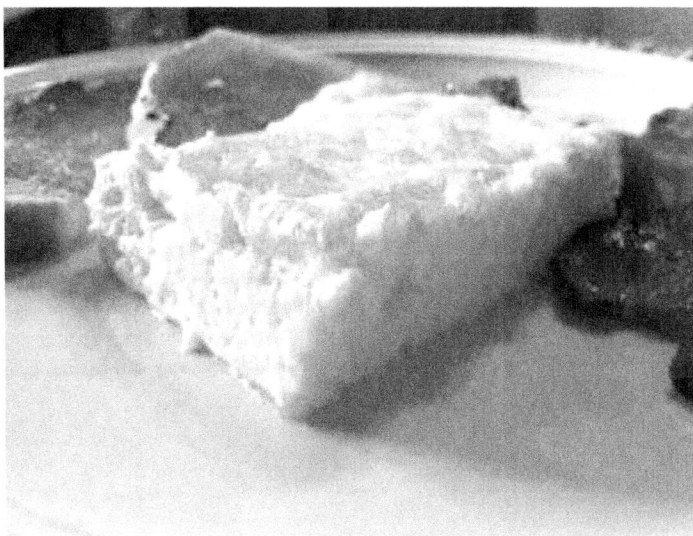

Directions:

1. Heat a skillet and melt the butter. Whisk the eggs with the cream cheese.
2. Cook until done. Serve.

Preparation time: 5 minutes

Cooking time: 5 minutes

Servings: 12

Ingredients:

- 3 lb. Italian sausage
- 8 oz. cream cheese
- 25 cup heavy cream
- 1/4 cup basil pesto
- 8 oz. mozzarella

Nutrition:

- Calories: 316
- Carbohydrates: 4 g
- Fat: 23 g
- Protein: 23 g

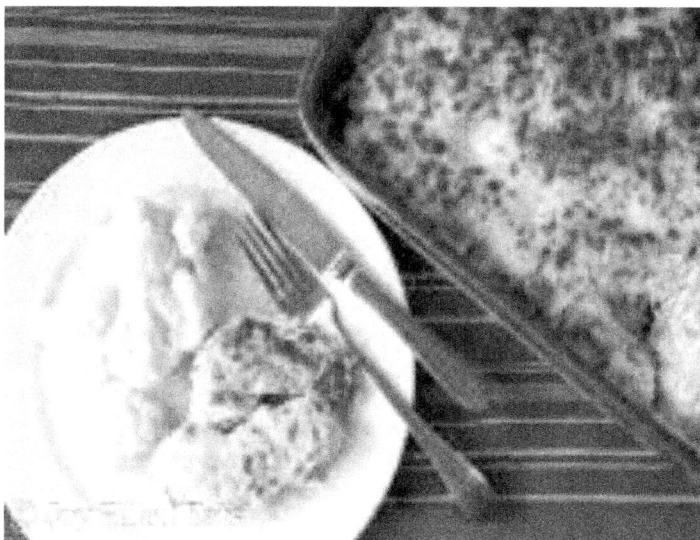

Directions:

1. Set the oven at 400°F.
2. Put the sausage in the dish and bake for 30 minutes. Combine the heavy cream, pesto, and cream cheese. Pour the sauce over the casserole and top it off with the cheese.
3. Bake for 10 minutes. Serve.

Preparation time: 5 minutes

Cooking time: 5 minutes

Servings: 4

Ingredients:

- 5 organic eggs
- 1 tbsp. coconut flour
- 1/4 tsp. sea salt
- 2 tbsp. almond meal

Nutrition:

- Calories: 111
- Carbohydrates: 3 g
- Fat: 8 g
- Protein: 8 g

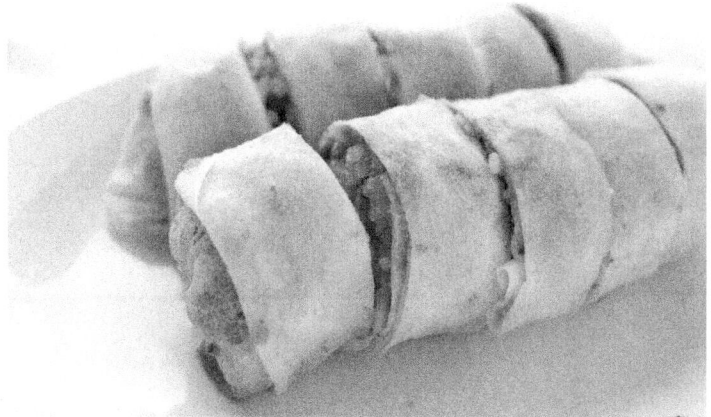

Directions:

1. Blend the ingredients in a blender. Warm-up a skillet, medium-high.
2. Put 2 tablespoons of the mixture then cook for 3 minutes.
3. Flip to cook for another 3 minutes. Serve.

Preparation time: 5 minutes

Cooking time: 2 minutes

Servings: 4

Ingredients:

- 1 cup almond flour
- 1 tsp. low carb baking powder
- 2 1/2 tbsp. swerve
- 1/3 tsp. salt
- 1 1/4 cup ricotta cheese
- 1/3 cup coconut milk
- 2 large eggs
- 1 cup heavy whipping cream

Nutrition:

- Calories: 407
- Carbohydrates: 7 g
- Fat: 31 g
- Protein: 12 g

Directions:

1. In a medium bowl, whisk the almond flour, baking powder, swerve, and salt. Set aside.
2. Then, crack the eggs into the blender and process them at medium speed for 30 seconds. Add the ricotta cheese, continue processing it, and gradually pour the coconut milk in while you keep on blending.
3. In about 90 seconds, the mixture will be creamy and smooth. Pour it into the dry ingredients and whisk to combine.
4. Set a skillet over medium heat and let it heat for a minute. Then, fetch a soup spoonful of mixture into the skillet and cook it for 1 minute.
5. Flip the pancake and cook further for 1 minute. Remove onto a plate and repeat the cooking process until the batter is xhausted. Serve the pancakes with whipping cream.

Preparation time: 5 minutes

Cooking time: 5 minutes

Servings: 1

Ingredients:

- 2 tbsp. ground coffee
- 1/3 cup heavy whipping cream
- 1 tsp. ground cinnamon
- 2 cups of water

Nutrition:

- Calories: 136
- Carbohydrates: 1 g
- Fiber: 1 g
- Fat: 14 g
- Protein: 1 g

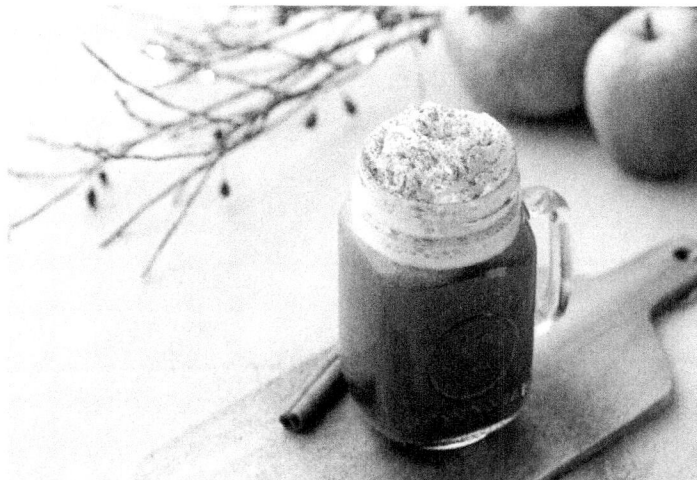

Directions:

1. Start by mixing the cinnamon with the ground coffee.
2. Pour in hot water, whip the cream until stiff peaks.
3. Serve with cinnamon.

Preparation time: 10
minutes

Cooking time: 0 minutes

Servings: 2

Ingredients:

- 1 vanilla shortbread
  collagen protein bar
- 1 tbsp. lemon
- 1/4 tsp. ground ginger
- 1/2 cup unsweetened
  coconut flakes
- 1/4 tsp. ground turmeric
- 1 spoon of water

Nutrition:

- Calories: 204
- Carbohydrates: 4.2 g
- Fat: 11 g
- Protein: 1.5 g

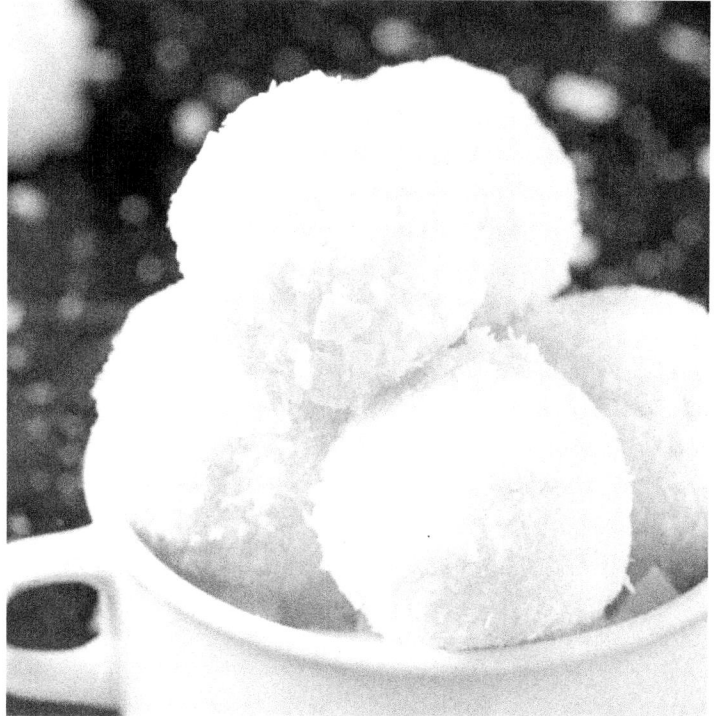

Directions:

1. Process protein bar, ginger, turmeric, and 3/4 of the total flakes into a food processor.
2. Remove and add 1 spoon of water and 1 tbsp. lemon and roll till dough forms.
3. Roll into balls and sprinkle the rest of the flakes on it. Serve.

Preparation time: 5 Minutes

Cooking time: 4 Minutes

Servings: 4

Ingredients:

- 2 oz. avocado smashed
- 2 slices of bread toasted
- A pinch of kosher salt and cracked black pepper
- 1/4 tsp. freshly squeezed lemon juice
- 2 eggs see notes, poached
- 3 1/2 oz. smoked salmon
- 1 tbsp. thinly sliced scallions
- Splash of Kikkoman soy sauce (optional)
- Microgreens are (optional)

Nutrition:

- Calories: 459
- Fat: 22 g
- Carbohydrates: 33 g
- Protein: 31 g

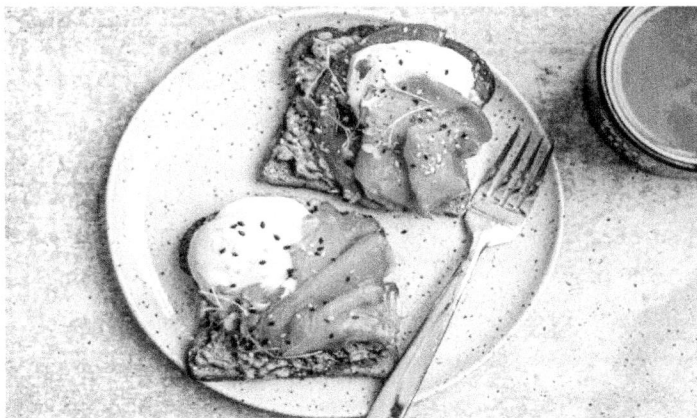

Directions:

1. Take a small bowl and then smash the avocado into it. Then, add the lemon juice and a pinch of salt into the mixture. Then, mix it well and set it aside.
2. After that, poach the eggs and toast the bread for some time.
3. Once the bread is toasted, you will have to spread the avocado on both slices and after that, add the smoked salmon to each slice.
4. Thereafter, carefully transfer the poached eggs to the respective toasts.
5. Add a splash of Kikkoman soy sauce and some cracked pepper; then, just garnish with scallions and microgreens.

Smoothies are great for breakfast on the go because they are quick, fill you up, and provide lasting energy throughout the morning.

Preparation time: 10 mins

Cooking time: 0 minutes

Servings: 2

Ingredients:

- 2 bananas, peeled
- 1 cup unsweetened almond milk, or skim milk
- 1 cup crushed ice
- 3 tbsp. unsweetened cocoa powder
- 3 tbsp. honey

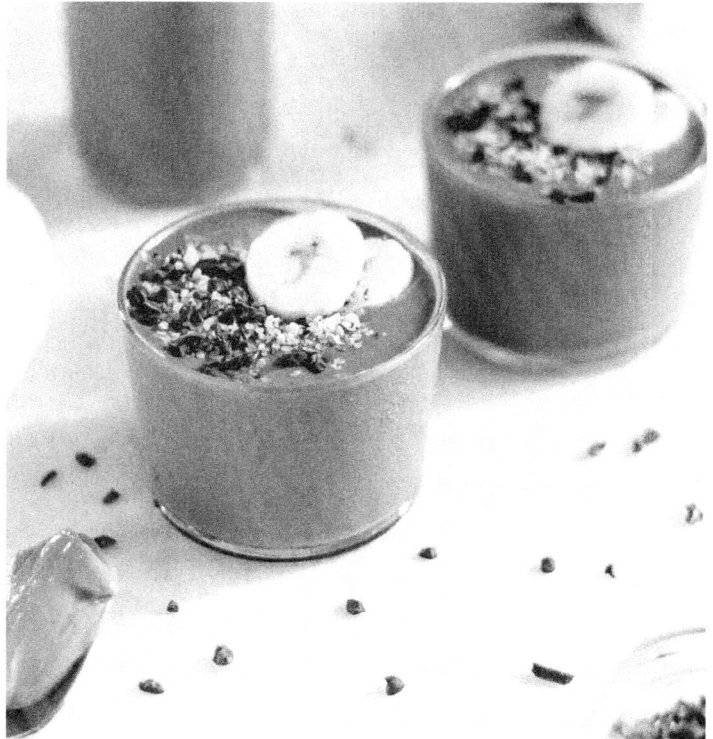

Nutrition:

- Calories: 246
- Carbohydrates: 24.5 g
- Fat: 11.1 g
- Fiber: 4.7 g
- Protein: 13.7 g

Directions:

1. In a blender, combine the bananas, almond milk, ice, cocoa powder, and honey.
2. Blend until smooth.
3. You can refrigerate leftovers and blend the next day for about 30 seconds at high speed.

Preparation time: 5 minutes

Cooking time: 5 minutes

Servings: 2

Ingredients:

- 2 cups blueberries (or any fresh or frozen fruit, cut into pieces if the fruit is large)
- 2 cups unsweetened almond milk
- 1 cup crushed ice
- 1/2 tsp. ground ginger (or other dried ground spice such as turmeric, cinnamon, or nutmeg)

Nutrition:

- Calories: 246
- Carbohydrates: 24.5 g
- Fat: 11.1 g
- Fiber: 4.7 g
- Protein: 13.7 g

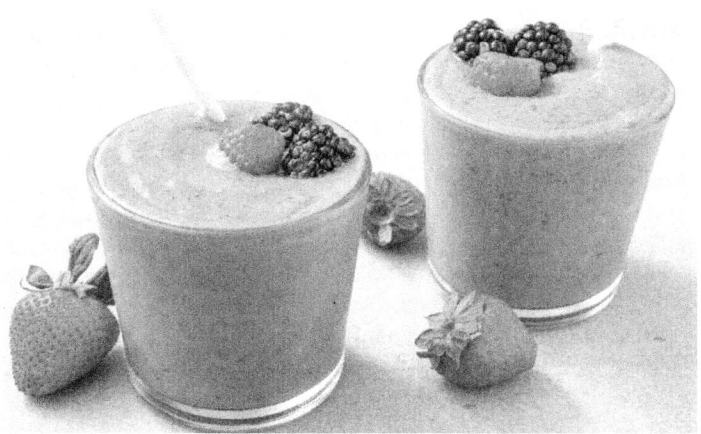

Directions:

1. In a blender, combine the blueberries, almond milk, ice, and ginger. Blend until smooth.
2. Some flavor combinations to try ginger and blueberry, honeydew melon and turmeric, mango and nutmeg, or mixed berries and cinnamon. Have fun experimenting

Note:

The great thing about fruit smoothies is how easy it is to customize them using seasonal produce. Because fruit is naturally sweet, you don't need to add any additional sweetener here. If using seasonal fruits, opt for fresh. In the absence of seasonal fruits, use frozen fruits.

Preparation time: 10 minutes

Cooking time: 0 minutes

Servings: 2

Ingredients:

- 1/2 cup vanilla low-fat Greek yogurt
- 1/4 cup low-fat milk
- 1/2 cup fresh or frozen blueberries or strawberries (or a combination)
- 6–8 ice cubes

Nutrition:

- Calories: 90
- Carbohydrates: 23.9 g
- Fat: 0.3 g
- Protein: 0.5 g

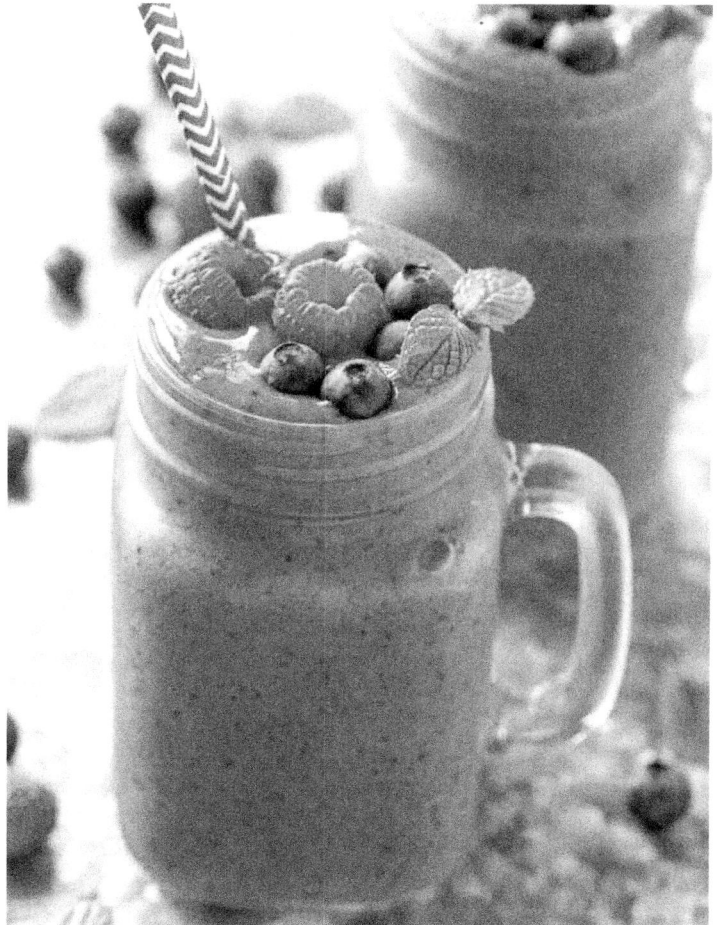

Directions:

1. Place the Greek yogurt, milk, and berries in a blender and blend until the berries are liquefied. Add the ice cubes and blend on high until thick and smooth. Serve immediately.

Preparation time: 8 minutes

Cooking time: 0 minutes

Servings: 2

Ingredients:

- 1 cup strawberries, fresh and sliced
- 1 rhubarb stalk, chopped
- 2 tbsp. honey, raw
- 3 ice cubes
- 1/8 tsp. ground cinnamon
- 1/2 cup Greek yogurt, plain
- Water

Nutrition:

- Calories: 295
- Fat: 8 g
- Carbohydrates: 56 g
- Protein: 6 g

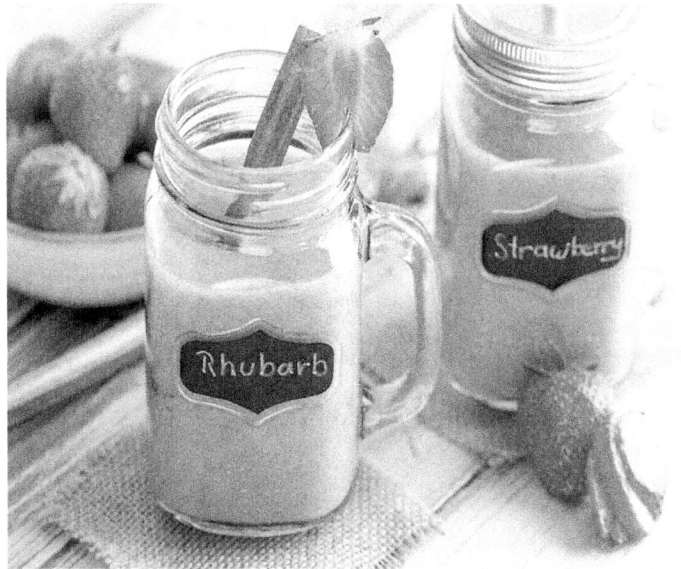

Directions:

1. Start by getting out a small saucepan and fill it with water. Place it over high heat to bring it to a boil, and then add in your rhubarb.
2. Boil for 3 minutes before draining and transferring it to a blender.
3. In your blender, add in your yogurt, honey, cinnamon, and strawberries. Blend until smooth, and then add in your ice.
4. Blend until there are no lumps and it's thick. Enjoy cold.

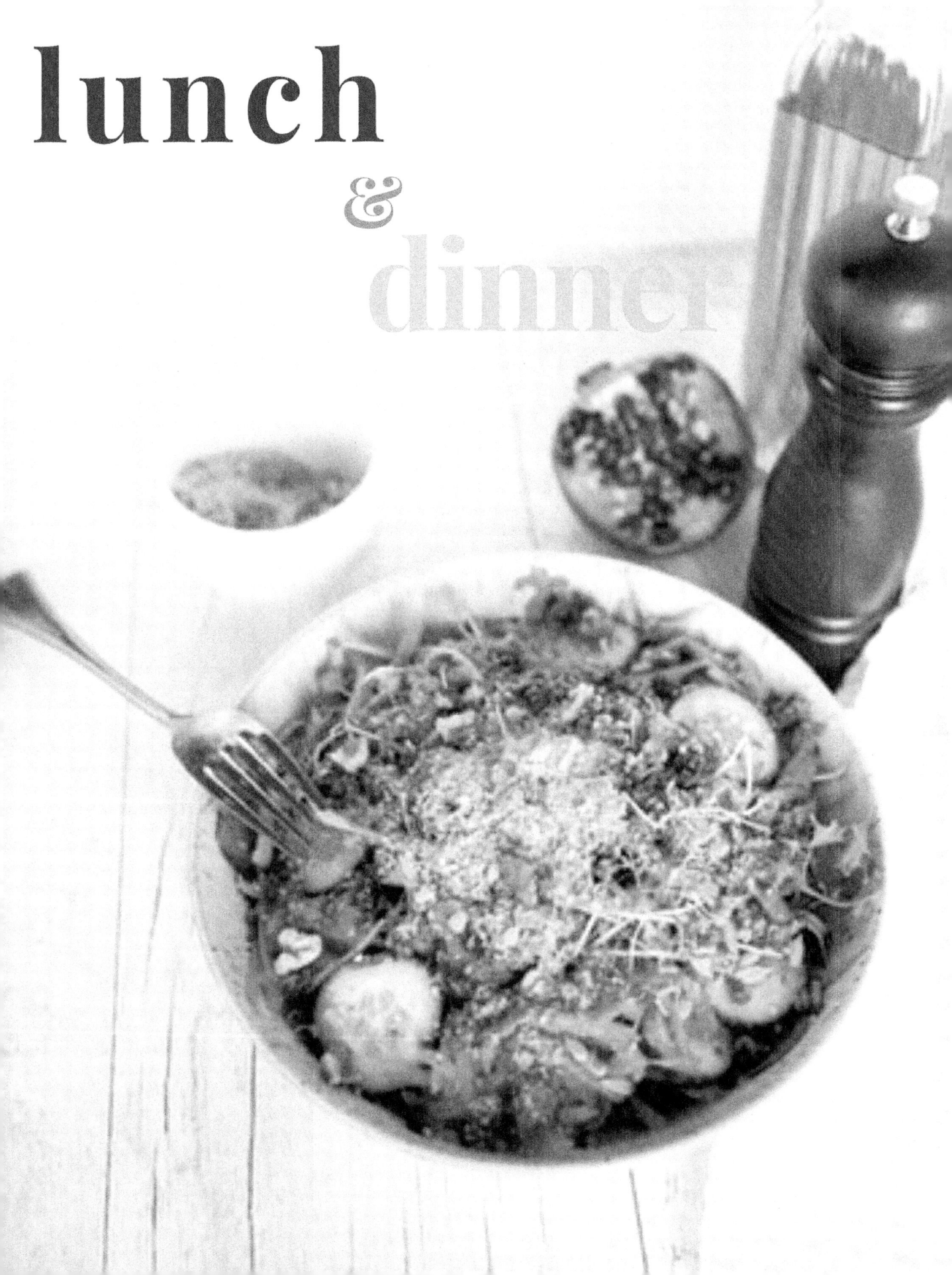

lunch
&
dinner

16. Cilantro Chicken Breasts with Mayo-Avocado Sauce

Preparation time: 5 minutes

Cooking time: 20 minutes

Servings: 4

Ingredients:

Mayo-avocado sauce:

- 1 avocado, pitted
- 1/2 cup mayonnaise
- Salt to taste

Chicken:

- 2 tbsp. ghee
- 4 chicken breasts
- Pink salt and black pepper to taste
- 2 tbsp. fresh cilantro, chopped
- 1/2 cup chicken broth

Nutrition:

- Calories: 398
- Fat: 32 g
- Carbohydrates: 4 g
- Protein 24 g

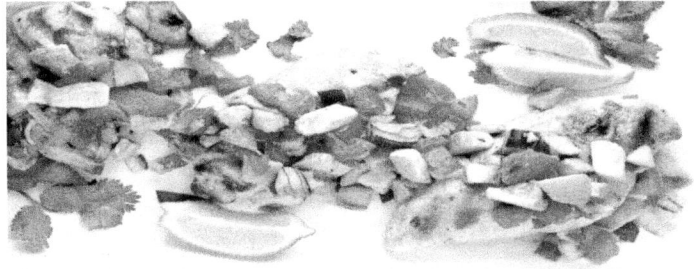

Directions:

1. Spoon the avocado into a bowl and mash with a fork. Add in mayonnaise and salt and stir until a smooth sauce is derived. Pour sauce into a jar and refrigerate. Melt the ghee in a large skillet over medium heat. Season chicken with salt and pepper and fry for 4 minutes on each side until golden brown.

2. Pour the broth in the same skillet and add the cilantro. Bring to simmer covered for 3 minutes and return the chicken. Cover and cook on low heat for 5 minutes until the liquid has reduced and the chicken is fragrant. Place the chicken only into serving plates and spoon the mayo-avocado sauce over. Serve.

Preparation time: 10 Mins

Cooking time: 15 Minutes

Servings: 4

Ingredients:

Skewers:

- 3 tbsp. soy sauce
- 1 tbsp. ginger-garlic paste
- 2 tbsp. swerve brown sugar
- 1 tsp. chili pepper
- 2 tbsp. olive oil
- 1 lb. chicken breasts, cut into cubes

Dressing

- 1/2 cup tahini
- 1/2 tsp. garlic powder
- Pink salt to taste
- 1/4 cup of warm water

Nutrition:

- Calories: 225
- Fat: 17.4 g
- Carbohydrates: 2 g
- Protein: 15 g

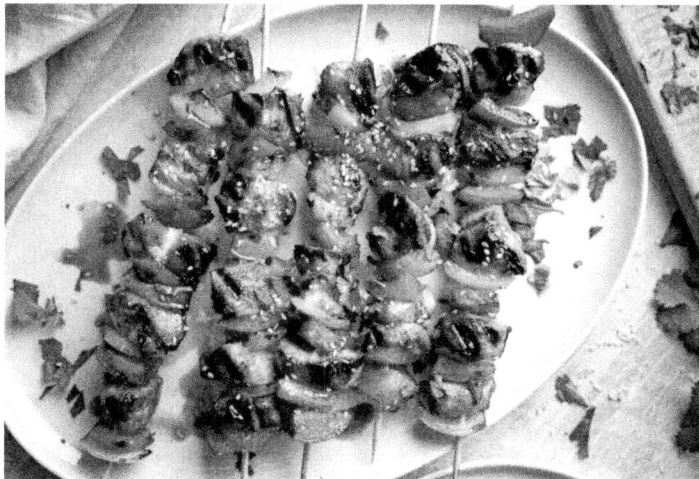

Directions:

1. In a bowl, whisk soy sauce, ginger-garlic paste, swerve brown sugar, chili pepper, and olive oil. Put the chicken in a zipper bag. Pour in the marinade, seal, and shake to coat. Marinate in the fridge for 2 hours.

2. Preheat grill to 400°F. Thread the chicken on skewers. Cook for 10 minutes in total with three to four turnings until golden brown; remove to a plate. Mix the tahini, garlic powder, salt, and 1/4 cup of warm water in a bowl. Pour into serving jars. Serve the chicken skewers and tahini dressing with Cauli rice.

Preparation time: 15 minutes

Cooking time: 30 minutes

Servings: 2

Ingredients:

- 1 tbsp. peanut oil or avocado oil, divided
- 4 oz. bacon, sliced thickly
- 1/2 cup red cabbage, finely shredded
- 2 garlic cloves, minced
- 1 tbsp. grated fresh ginger root
- 1/4 tsp. crushed red pepper flakes, or to taste (optional)
- 2 tsp. dark sesame oil, divided
- 1/4 cup coconut Aminos or low sodium soy sauce

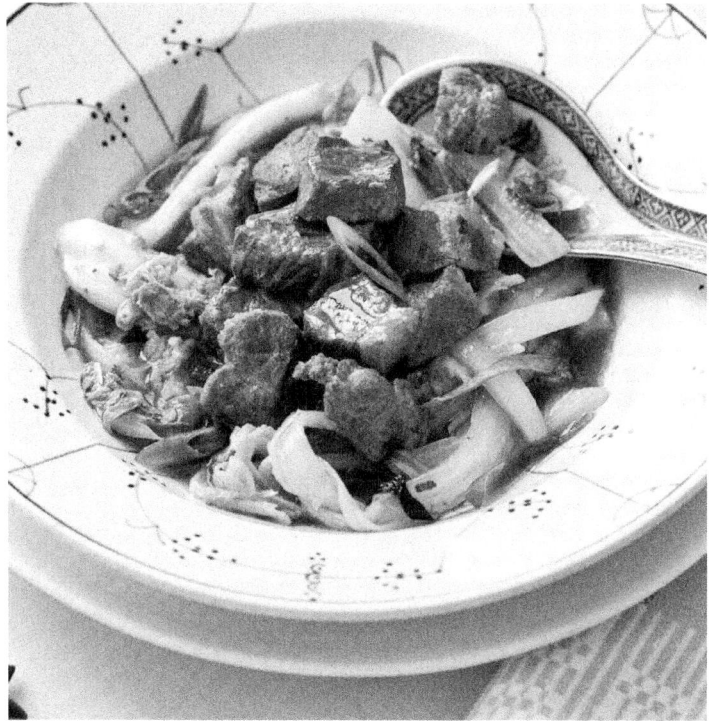

Directions:

1. Heat 1 tsp. peanut oil in a large, deep skillet over high heat. Add the bacon and cook until crispy. Transfer to a bowl and set aside.
2. Add the remaining oil to the skillet and then add half the red cabbage. Cook, stirring often, until wilted-about 3 minutes, then transfer to a large bowl.
3. Add the garlic, ginger root, and red pepper flakes to the skillet; cook 1 minute over

Nutrition:

- Calories: 76
- Fat: 5 g
- Carbohydrates: 3 g
- Fiber: 1 g
- Sugar: 0 g
- Protein: 5 g

medium-low heat. Stir in half the sesame oil and stir in enough of the bacon drippings or other fat to coat the pan. Cook 3 minutes over medium-low heat for a slightly thickened sauce.

4. Stir in the cabbage, bacon, coconut Aminos, and soy sauce. Cook until the cabbage is heated through, and the sauce has thickened about 7 minutes. This should be done over low heat, so you don't overcook the cabbage. Transfer to a serving bowl and sprinkle with remaining sesame oil before serving with steamed white rice or your favorite grain.

Preparation time: 15 mins

Cooking time: 45 minutes

Servings: 2

Ingredients:

- 16 oz. ricotta cheese, divided
- 1 tbsp. dried Italian seasoning, divided
- 2 tbsp. grated Parmesan cheese, divided
- 2/3 cup low-fat cottage cheese
- 1 large egg plus 3 egg whites, lightly beaten (or 2 whole eggs)
- 5 cups chopped zucchini
- 1 1/2 cups jarred tomato sauce
- 2 cups shredded mozzarella cheese, divided
- Cooking spray

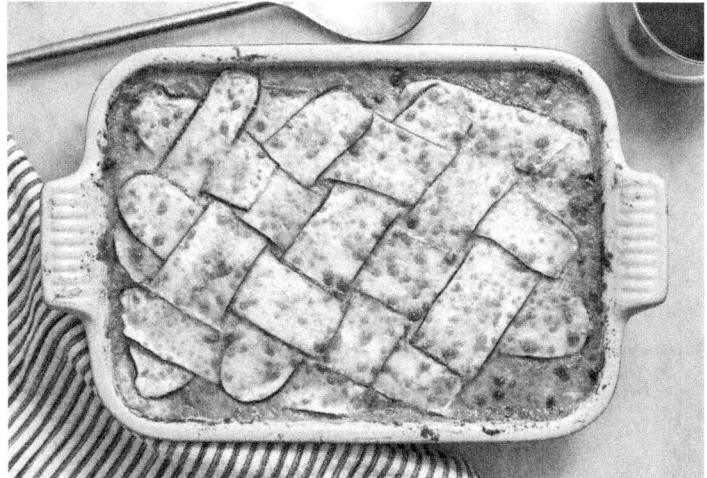

Directions:

1. Preheat oven to 400°F. Coat a 9-by-13-inch baking dish with nonstick cooking spray. Set aside. In a medium bowl, stir together 1/3 cup of the ricotta cheese, 1 tsp. of Italian seasoning, and 1 tsp. of Parmesan cheese; set aside. In another bowl, combine cottage cheese, egg, and egg whites, season with salt and pepper if desired. To make the lasagna rolls, layout flat about 5 sheets of lasagna noodles (3 to 4 inches wide) at a time on your countertop. Spoon about a quarter of the cottage cheese mixture in a line down the middle of the lasagna sheets, being careful

- Salt and pepper to taste
- 5 sheets of lasagna noodles

Nutrition:

- Calories: 208
- Fat: 10.6 g
- Carbohydrates: 12.1 g
- Fiber: 2.3 g
- Sugar: 4.7 g
- Protein: 16.2 g

not to spread it out. Sprinkle a small amount of mozzarella cheese, zucchini, and tomato sauce over the cottage cheese mixture. Then evenly lay out more lasagna sheets on top of this (about 5 or 6 sheets) and fold over the ends to cover it.

2. Roll up the lasagna sheet with the cottage cheese mixture in it like you would roll up a jelly roll and transfer it to an ungreased baking dish seam side down. Repeat for all remaining ingredients to create 3 more rolls in total. Cover the baking dish with aluminum foil and bake at 400°F for 45 minutes. Remove the foil and cover the dish again for 15 more minutes. Transfer to a serving plate, slice into 6 portions and sprinkle with remaining leftover Parmesan cheese.

Preparation time: 10 mins

Cooking time: 15 minutes

Servings: 2

Ingredients:

- 12 oz. flank steak, cut into bite-sized pieces
- 6 tbsp. butter, divided
- 4 garlic cloves, minced, divided
- 1 tsp. paprika, divided
- 3 cups baby arugula or spinach salad mix (about 1 oz.)
- 1 cup cherry tomatoes, halved or quartered if large
- 1/4 cup crumbled blue cheese (optional)
- Salt and pepper to taste

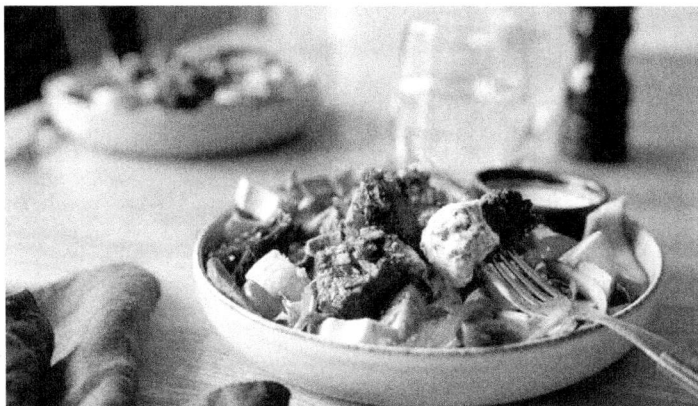

Directions:

1. In a small bowl add 1 tbsp. of the minced garlic and 2 tsp. paprika; set aside. Heat 2 tbsp. butter over medium-high heat in a large skillet for 30 seconds. Add the steak and season with salt and pepper; cook 6 minutes, tossing frequently to brown evenly on both sides. Transfer the steak to a plate. Add the remaining 2 tbsp. butter and the remaining 4 garlic cloves to the pan; cook 1 minute over medium heat.

2. Add the steak back into the pan with any juices that have accumulated on the plate, season with salt and pepper if desired. Lower heat to medium-low and stir in garlic-paprika mixture, cooking for an additional

Nutrition:

- Calories: 214
- Fat: 15 g
- Carbohydrates: 3 g
- Fiber: 2 g
- Sugar: 0.5 g
- Protein: 15.5 g

minute until fragrant. Pour into a large bowl and add arugula or spinach, tomatoes, and blue cheese if using. Toss until combined. Serve immediately or refrigerate for later use as it tastes best when eaten cold.

Preparation time: 15 mis

Cooking time: 20-30 mins

Servings: 2

Ingredients:

- 1 tsp. coconut oil, divided
- 1 lb. ground pork sausage (80/20)
- 1/2 tsp. ground nutmeg, divided
- 1 small onion, diced small (about 1/4 cup)
- 4 cups pumpkin puree (canned or fresh)
- 4 cups chicken broth
- 1 cup heavy whipping cream or coconut milk
- 2 tbsp. fresh sage, minced
- Salt and freshly ground black pepper to taste

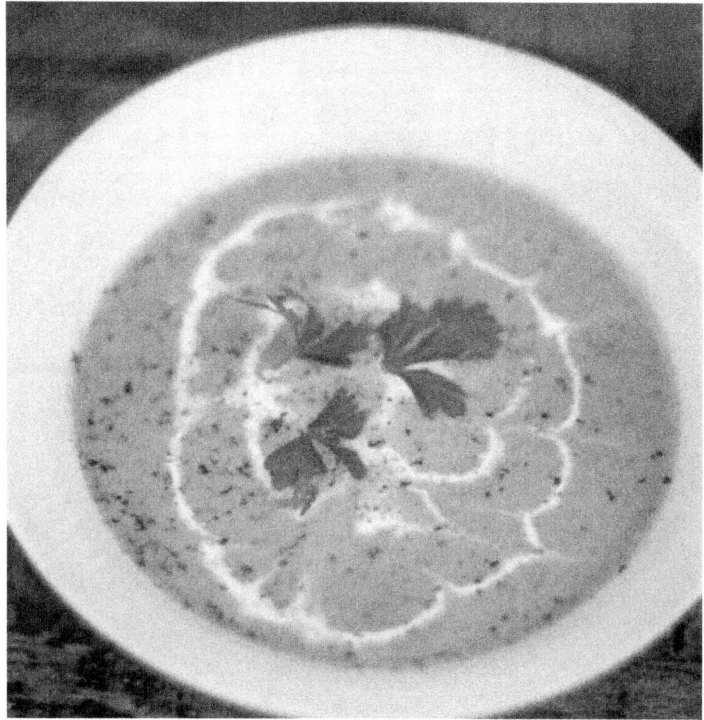

Directions:

1. Heat 1 tsp. of the oil in a medium saucepan over medium-high heat and add the sausage. Cook until well browned, stirring occasionally for about 10 minutes. Transfer sausage to a plate with a slotted spoon and set aside. Add the nutmeg to the sausage drippings in the saucepan; cook over low heat for 1 minute until fragrant, stirring constantly. Add the onion and cook 6

Nutrition:

- Calories: 116
- Fat: 4 g
- Carbohydrates: 6.5 g
- Fiber: 2.6 g
- Sugar: 3 g
- Protein: 12.7 g

minutes until translucent, stirring frequently.

2. Add the remaining 1 tsp. oil to the saucepan; stir in pumpkin, broth, and cream, and bring to a simmer. Simmer for 4 minutes, stirring occasionally. Add the browned sausage with any juices back into the pot and stir well until well blended. Place mixture in a blender or food processor and blend until smooth, adding a little water, if needed. Stir in sage, salt and pepper then place back into the saucepan over medium heat; cook for 5 to 10 minutes until warm.

Preparation time: 15 mins

Cooking time: 50 to 60 mins

Servings: 2

Ingredients:

- 1 small yellow onion, chopped
- 2 garlic cloves, minced
- 1 tbsp. olive oil
- 3/4 cup chicken broth or water (or more if needed)
- 4 cups fresh baby spinach
- 2 Tomatoes
- Salt and pepper to taste
- 3 lb. pork shoulder

Nutrition:

- Calories: 438
- Fat: 28 g
- Carbohydrates: 2.4 g

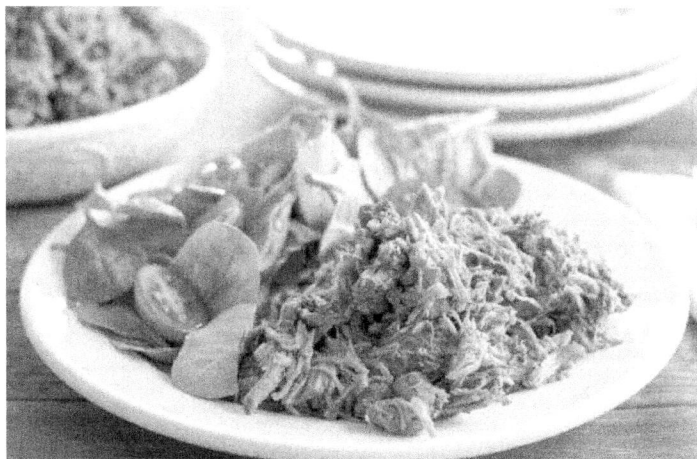

Directions:

1. Heat oven to 425°F. Wash the tomatoes. Cut the tops off and slice them in half lengthwise. Remove the seeds and sprinkle with salt and pepper. Put on a baking sheet and drizzle with olive oil, then roast for 20 minutes until soft. Using the same pan from roasting tomatoes, add olive oil over medium-high heat in a large skillet. Add whichever protein you choose into your skillet (in this recipe, I used a 3 lb. pork shoulder roast). Cook until browned evenly, breaking up the meat with a wooden spoon. Add 1 chopped onion into the skillet and cook for 4 to 5 minutes. Add the garlic and broth/water; reduce heat to

- Fiber: 0.4 g
- Sugar: 0.5 g
- Protein: 51.5 g

low and simmer for another 6 to 8 minutes or until meat is cooked through. Transfer meat to a large bowl and set aside. In a large skillet, add remaining onions, spinach leaves and drizzle with olive oil. Season with salt and pepper if desired. Cook over medium heat for 2 to 3 minutes until wilted yet still bright green in color (adjust cooking time as needed). Serve the pulled pork with roasted tomatoes and spinach salad.

Preparation time: 15 mins

Cooking time: 15 to 20 mins

Servings: 2

Ingredients:

- 4 large collard green leaves, washed and blotted dry (2 heaping cups)
- 4 oz. cooked wild salmon (about 3/4 cup)
- 1/2 cup of chopped fresh cilantro
- 1/2 cup chopped fresh basil or mint or both
- 1/2 cup spinach
- 1/2 tsp. paprika, divided
- 1/4 tsp. crushed red chili pepper flakes, divided
- Salt and freshly ground black pepper to taste
- Juice of 1 lime (about 1 tbsp.)

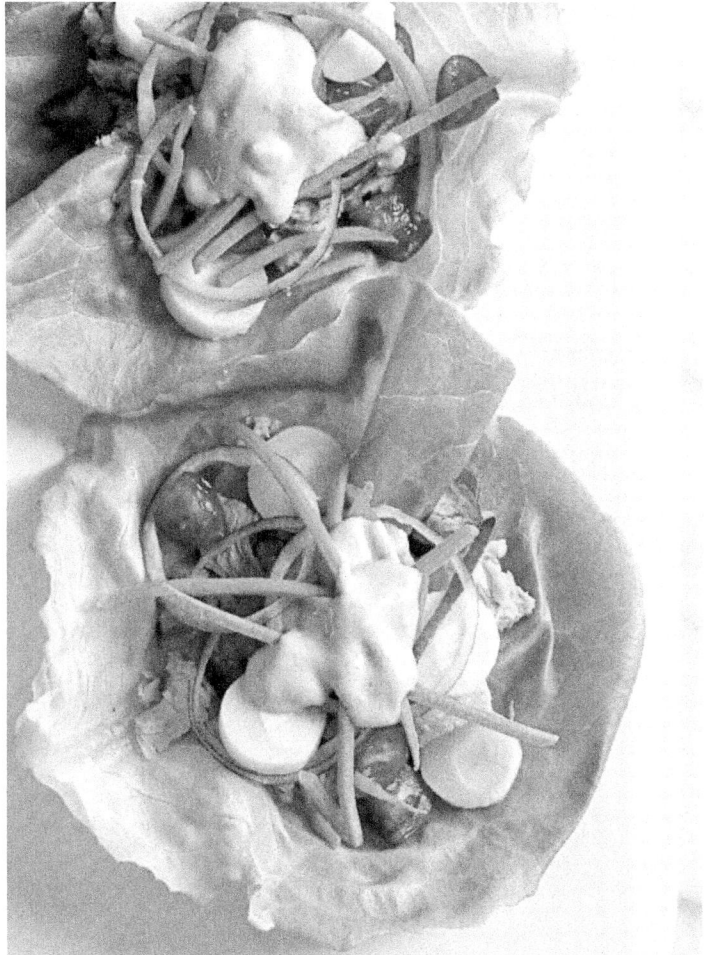

Directions:

1. Place a large skillet over medium-high heat. Add the olive oil into the skillet; swirl it around to coat. Add the tuna and season with salt, chili pepper, and paprika. Cook for about 3 minutes, tossing occasionally until

- 1 tbsp. olive oil or avocado oil (add more if needed)

Nutrition:

- Calories: 160
- Fat: 16 g
- Carbohydrates: 3 g
- Fiber: 1.5 g
- Sugar: 1 g
- Protein: 23.5 g

tuna is heated all the way through. Transfer tuna to a large bowl, then add spinach, basil or mint, cilantro, and lime juice to the bowl. Season with salt and pepper if desired. Toss until well blended then divide the mixture between the collard leaves; fold as needed to wrap them up. Serve with additional lime juice if desired. (Or shrimp or chicken for variation)

Preparation time: 10 Mins

Cooking time: 15 Mins

Servings: 8

Ingredients:

- 4 chicken breasts
- 4 slices of bacon
- 1/4 medium onion
- 2 garlic cloves
- 1/4 cup (60 ml) avocado oil, to cook with

Nutrition:

- Calories: 319
- Fat: 24 g
- Carbohydrates: 1 g
- Protein: 25 g

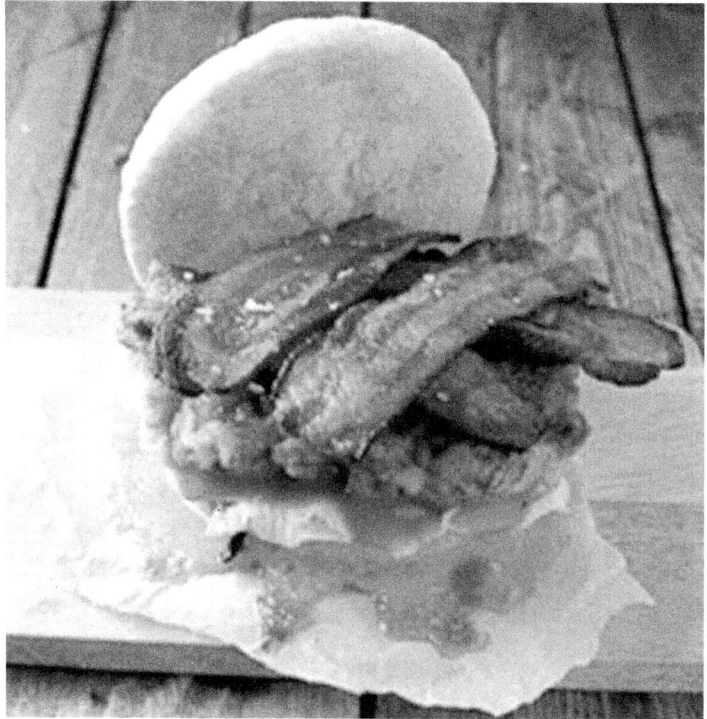

Directions:

1. Food process the chicken, bacon, onion, and garlic and form 8 patties. You need to do this in batches.
2. Fry patties in the avocado oil in batches. Make sure burgers are fully cooked.
3. Serve with guacamole.

Preparation time: 15 mins

Cooking time: 20 to 25 mins

Servings: 2

Ingredients:

- 1 lb. firm white fish fillets (salmon or cod work best)
- 1 tsp. salt, divided
- 1/2 tsp. freshly ground black pepper, divided
- 1 cup cooked quinoa
- 2 scallions, thinly sliced (about 1/3 cup)
- Salt and freshly ground black pepper to taste
- Cooking spray
- 1 zucchini
- Oil to taste

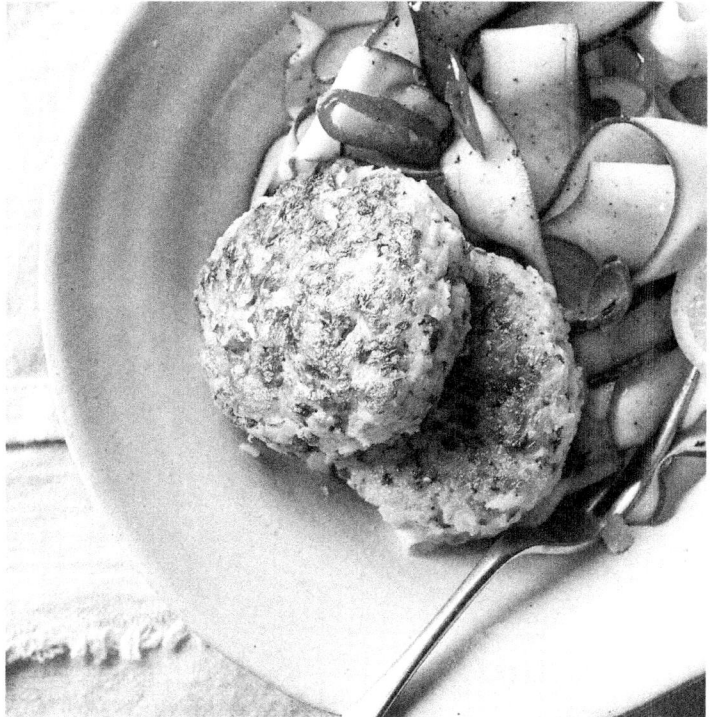

Directions:

1. Heat oven to 400°F then lines a baking sheet with parchment paper. Wash and pat dry the zucchini then cut into 1/4-inch-thick slices. Arrange slices in a single layer on the baking sheet then sprinkle with salt. Bake for 10 minutes until tender but still firm; set aside. Line a second baking sheet with aluminum foil and spray generously with nonstick cooking spray. Season the fish with 1 tsp. salt

Nutrition:

- Calories: 135
- Fat: 4 g
- Carbohydrates: 6 g
- Fiber: 1.5 g
- Sugar: 0.5 g
- Protein: 17.5 g

and 1/4 tsp. pepper. Heat a large skillet such as cast iron on medium heat and add enough oil to coat the bottom. Add the fish then cook for about 2 minutes, turning once. Transfer to the prepared baking sheet and continue with the remaining fish; cook in batches as needed.

2. Toast quinoa according to package directions and set aside until ready to use; set aside until "topping."

3. Heat broiler or grill (no oil required) and line a baking sheet with foil. Divide fish cakes between 4 bowls (about 1 1/2 tbsp. each); top each bowl with a spoonful of quinoa, zucchini than a sprinkle of scallions then remaining salt and pepper. Broil or grill fishcakes for 3 to 5 minutes until browned and heated through.

Preparation time: 10 Mins

Cooking time: 20 Minutes

Servings: 4

Ingredients:

- 1 lb. grass-fed lamb
- 1/4 cup chives finely chopped green onion or red onion if desired
- 1 tbsp. chopped fresh dill
- 1/2 tsp. dried oregano or about 1 tbsp. freshly chopped
- 1 tbsp. finely chopped fresh mint
- A pinch of chopped red pepper
- Fine-grained sea salt to taste
- 1 tbsp. water
- 2 tsp. olive oil to grease the pan

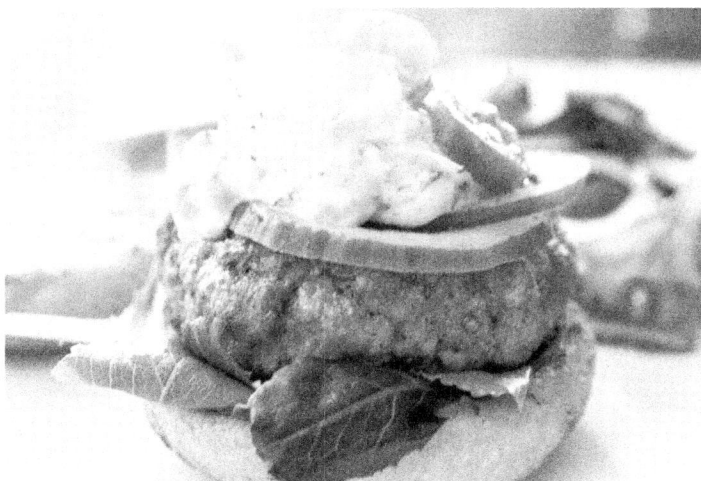

Directions:

1. Place the garlic, cucumber, and lemon juice in the food processor and press until finely chopped. Add the coconut cream, dill, salt, and pepper, and mix until well blended.
2. Put it in a jar with a lid and keep it in the refrigerator until it is served. The flavors become more intense over time when they cool in the fridge.
3. Thoroughly mix the ground lamb in a bowl with the chives or red onion, dill, oregano, mint, red pepper, and water.
4. Sprinkle the mixture with fine-grained sea salt and form 4 patties of the same size.

For the Tzatziki:

- 1 can coconut milk with all the cooled fat and 1 tbsp. the discarded liquid portion
- 3 garlic cloves
- 1 peeled cucumber without seeds, roughly sliced
- 1 tbsp. freshly squeezed lemon juice
- 2 tbsp. chopped fresh dill
- 3/4 tsp. fine grain sea salt
- Black pepper to taste

Nutrition:

- Calories: 363
- Fat: 22.14 g
- Carbohydrates: 6.83 g
- Protein: 35.33 g

5. Heat a large cast-iron skillet over medium heat and brush with a small amount of olive oil. Lightly sprinkle the pan with fine-grain sea salt.
6. Bring the patties into the pan and cook on each side for about 4 minutes, adjusting the heat to prevent the outside from becoming too brown. Alternatively, you can grill the burgers.
7. Remove from the pan and cover with Tzatziki sauce.

Preparation time: 5 Minutes

Cooking time: 15 Minutes

Servings: 6

Ingredients:

- 1 lb. minced lamb or half veal, half lamb
- 1/2 sliced onion
- 2 garlic cloves minced
- 1 tbsp. dried dill
- 1 tsp. salt
- 1/2 tsp. black pepper

Nutrition:

- Calories: 207
- Fat: 11.89 g
- Carbohydrates: 1.17 g
- Protein: 22.68 g

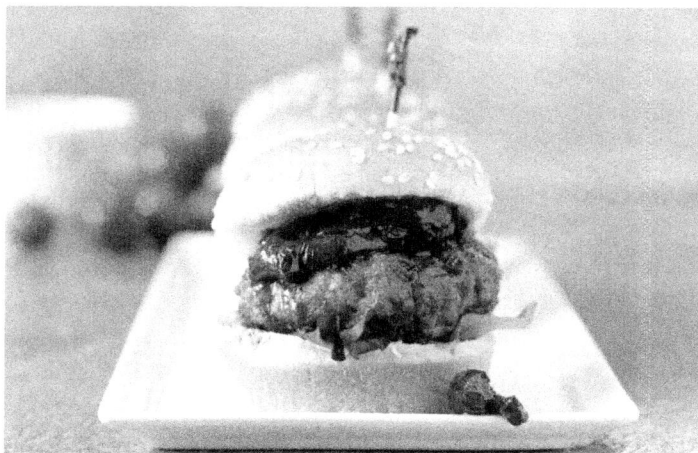

Directions:

1. Blend the ingredients gently in a large bowl until well combined. Overworking the meat will cause it to be tough.
2. Form the meat into burgers.
3. Grill or fry in a pan on medium-high heat until cooked through, 4 to 5 minutes per side. If preparing in a pan, sear both sides quickly, then throw the burgers in a 350°F oven for 10 minutes to finish cooking through.
4. Serve with Tzatziki for dipping!

Preparation time: 10 minutes

Cooking time: 25 to 30 minutes

Servings: 2

Ingredients:

- 1 tbsp. butter or ghee
- 1/2 cup prepared cream cheese or full-fat mozzarella
- 1/4 tsp. salt, divided
- 1/4 tsp. freshly ground black pepper, divided
- 1/8 tsp. dried thyme, divided
- 4 oz. of your favorite ground meat (ground turkey or beef are good choices)
- 4 oz. Mushrooms

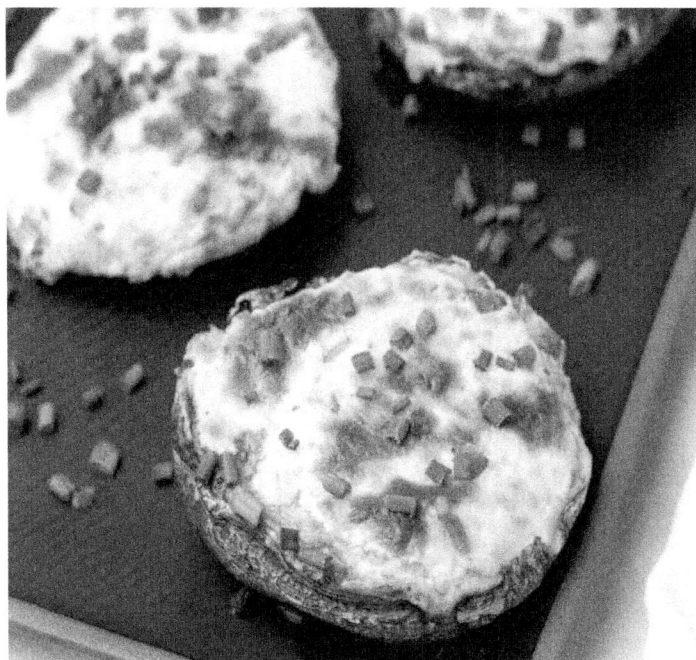

Directions:

1. Heat oven to 375°F. Melt butter/ghee in a small skillet over medium heat, then add mushrooms; sauté for 2 to 3 minutes. Add in the cream cheese, salt, pepper, and thyme; mix to combine. Stuff mushrooms with the mixture and transfer to a baking sheet lined with parchment paper, then drizzle with olive oil (if desired). Bake for 10 minutes until mushrooms are tender and cream cheese is softened; set aside.

Nutrition:

- Calories: 120
- Fat: 7 g
- Carbohydrates: 3 g
- Fiber: 0.5 g
- Sugar: 1 g
- Protein: 10 g

2. Heat a large skillet such as cast iron over medium heat then add the meat to the pan. Cook for about 5 minutes or until browned then season with remaining salt and pepper if desired.

3. Serve immediately with grilled vegetables or salad as desired. (Optional: top with additional mozzarella.)

Preparation time: 14 Mins

Cooking time: 6 Minutes

Servings: 4

Ingredients:

- 1 tbsp. olive oil
- 1 tsp. chili powder
- 2 tilapia fillets
- 1 tsp. paprika
- 4 low carb tortillas

Slaw:

- 1/2 cup red cabbage, shredded
- 1 tbsp. lemon juice
- 1 tsp. apple cider vinegar
- 1 tbsp. olive oil
- Salt and black pepper to taste

Directions:

1. Season the tilapia with chili powder and paprika. Heat the vegetable oil over a skillet over medium heat.
2. Add tilapia and cook until blackened, about 3 minutes per side. Cut into strips. Divide the tilapia between the tortillas. Blend all the slaw ingredients in a bowl and top the fish to serve.

Nutrition:

- Calories: 268
- Fat: 20 g
- Carbohydrates: 3.5 g
- Protein: 13.8 g

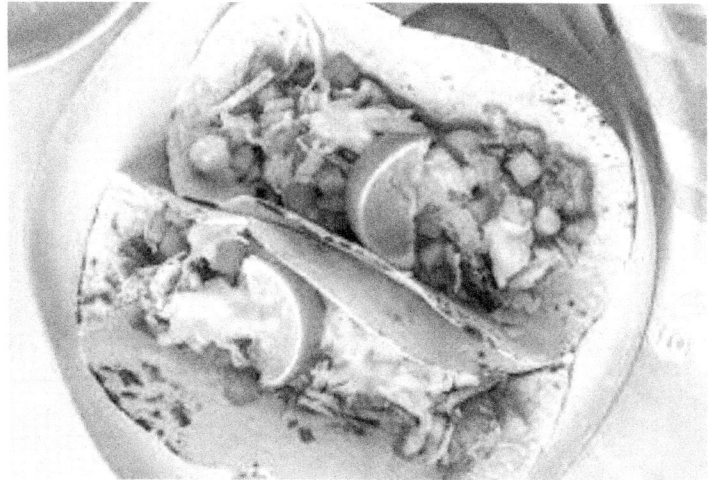

Preparation time: 10 mins

Cooking time: 15-20 minutes

Servings: 2

Ingredients:

- 1 tbsp. olive oil (optional)
- 2 tbsp. lemon zest, freshly squeezed (about 2 lemons)
- 1/4 cup fresh lemon juice, divided
- 4 oz. fish fillets (cod or salmon is best)
- 1/2 tsp. salt, divided
- 1/8 tsp. freshly ground black pepper, divided
- 4 green onions, thinly sliced (about 1/2 cup)

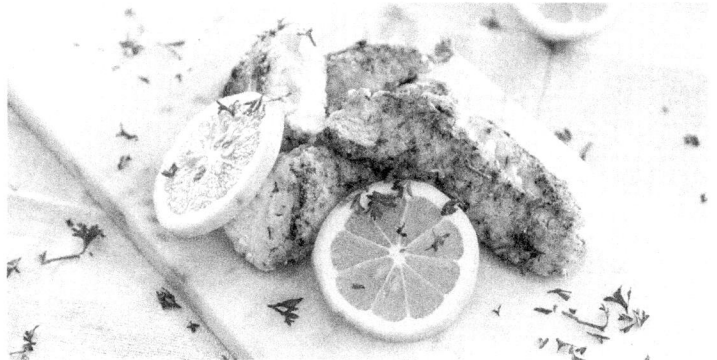

Directions:

1. Heat the oil in a large skillet over medium-high heat then add lemon zest and sauté for about 2 minutes. Add fish to the pan and season with salt, pepper, and lemon juice. Cover with a lid or aluminum foil. Cook for about four minutes or until the fish is white then turn off the heat. Add in green onions and serve immediately.

Nutrition:

- Calories: 125
- Fat: 6 g
- Carbohydrates: 3 g
- Fiber: 0.5 g
- Sugar: 1 g
- Protein: 13 g

Preparation time: 10 Mins

Cooking time: 15 Minutes

Servings: 4

Ingredients:

Salmon skewers:

- 60 ml finely chopped fresh basil
- 450 g salmon
- Salt and black pepper to taste
- 100 g dried ham sliced
- 1 tbsp. olive oil
- 8 pieces wooden skewers
- Water

Innings:

- 225 ml mayonnaise

Nutrition:

- Calories: 680
- Carbohydrates: 1 g
- Fats: 62 g
- Proteins: 28 g

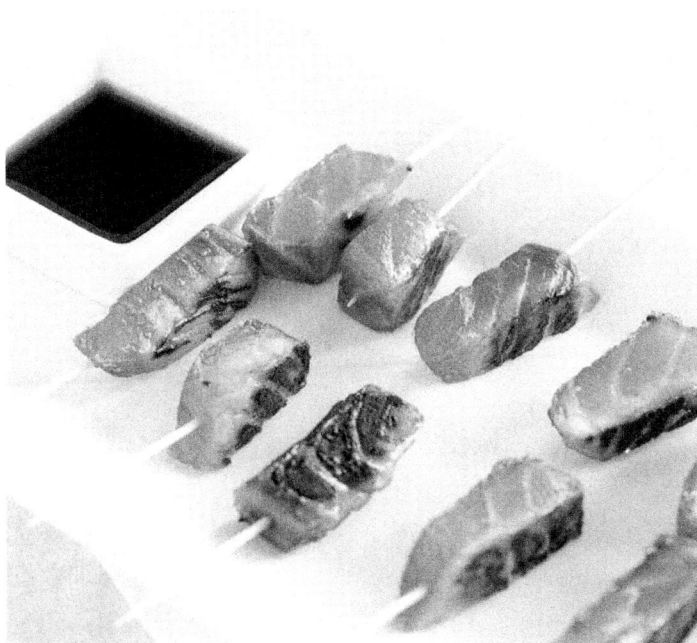

Directions:

1. Soak the skewers in water.
2. Finely chop fresh basil.
3. Cut salmon fillet into rectangular pieces and fasten-on skewers.
4. Roll each kebab in the basil and pepper.
5. Cut the cured ham into thin slices and wrap her every kebab.
6. Sprinkle with olive oil and fry in a pan, grill, or in the oven.
7. Serve with mayonnaise or salad

Preparation time: 15 mins

Cooking time: 15 to 20 mins

Servings: 2

Ingredients:

- 1 1/2 lb. cod fillets, skinned
- 2 pinches ground black pepper, divided
- 2 pinches fresh grated nutmeg, divided
- 1/2 tsp. salt, divided
- 1/4 cup butter or ghee (1/4 stick), grated and at room temperature
- 4 oz. of your favorite horseradish sauce (about 1/3 cup)
- 2 tbsp. heavy cream or half-and-half (optional)

Nutrition:

- Calories: 295
- Fat: 16 g
- Carbohydrates: 4 g
- Fiber: 1 g
- Sugar: 0.5 g
- Protein: 31 g

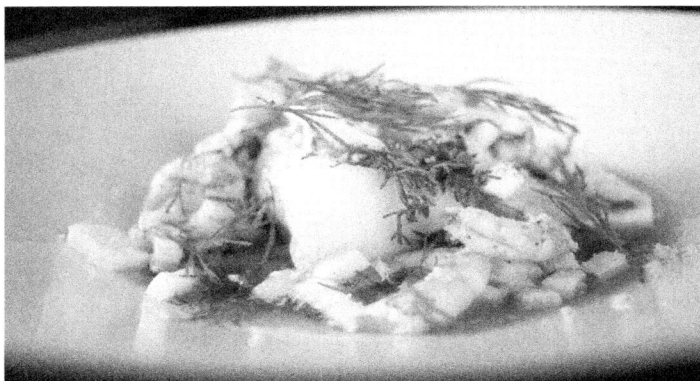

Directions:

1. Heat oven to 375°F then arranges a baking sheet with parchment paper. Rinse the fish and pat dry with paper towels. Season with pepper and nutmeg; drizzle with butter, then season again with salt. Arrange a layer of fish on the baking sheet then sprinkle with one pinch of salt and one pinch of pepper. Continue until all fish is in the pan. Bake for about 15 to 20 minutes or until fish flakes when tested with a fork; set aside.

2. Heat oven to 450°F then adds the butter to a small skillet over medium heat. Cook butter until browned and bubbly. Add horseradish sauce then cream (if desired) to the pan; stir together until hot and well combined in an even sauce. Serve cod fillets with the sauce drizzled over top, garnished with additional nutmeg if desired.

Preparation time: 10 mins

Cooking time: 20-30 minutes

Servings: 2

Ingredients:

- 1 medium onion, diced
- 2 celery stalks, diced
- 2 tbsp. butter or ghee
- 1 cup heavy cream or half-and-half (optional)
- 1/2 cup clam juice (about 2 cans)
- 2 cups chicken stock or chicken broth (about 8 oz.)
- 4 oz. cooked shrimp (about 1 1/2 cups)
- Sea salt and freshly ground black pepper to taste
- 2 inches of water

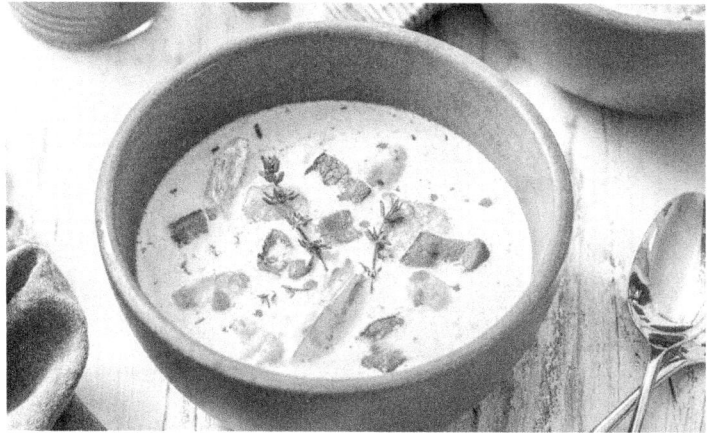

Nutrition:

- Calories: 181
- Fat: 12 g
- Carbohydrates: 5 g
- Fiber: 0.5 g
- Sugar: 3 g
- Protein: 9 g

Directions:

1. Heat a large pot with about 2 inches of water over medium heat then add onions and celery; cook for about five minutes until softened then add in the butter/ghee. Cook for another minute then pour in heavy cream/half-and-half and clam juice; bring to a boil. Add the broth and shrimp, then reduce heat to a simmer; cook for about 15 minutes or until seafood is cooked through. Season with salt and pepper as desired, then serve immediately.

Preparation time: 25 mins

Servings: 2

Ingredients:

- 4 tbsp. butter or ghee, melted
- 1/2 lb. tilapia fillet, thawed and cut into bite-size pieces
- 1 medium red bell pepper, chopped (optional)
- Sea salt and freshly ground black pepper to taste
- Parmesan cheese to taste
- Parsley to taste
- Lemon slices to taste

Nutrition:

- Calories: 296
- Fat: 18 g
- Carbohydrates: 2.6 g
- Fiber: 0 g
- Sugar: 0 g
- Protein: 26.4 g

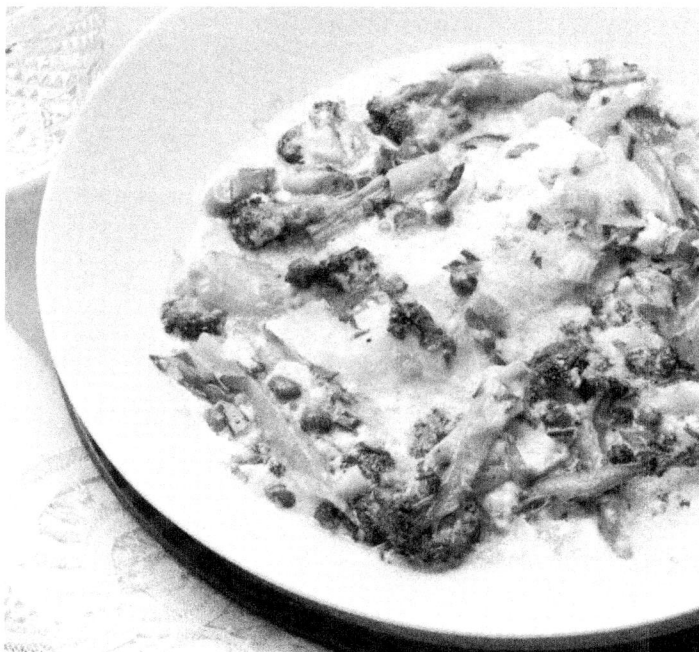

Directions:

1. Preheat oven to 350°F. Combine butter and seasonings in a small bowl; place on the fish pieces, coating thoroughly. Arrange fish in an 8x11 or 9x13 baking dish; bake for about 15 minutes until cooked through. Alternatively, you can broil for about 5 minutes or until lightly golden browned. Remove from heat and top with Parmesan cheese, parsley and lemon slices; serve immediately.

Preparation time: 10 Mins

Cooking time: 10 Minutes

Servings: 2

Ingredients:

- 1 cup avocado oil or coconut oil, plus more as needed
- 1 lb. frozen mahi-mahi, thawed
- 2 large eggs
- 2 tbsp. avocado oil mayonnaise
- 1 cup almond flour
- 1/2 cup shredded coconut
- 1/4 cup crushed macadamia nuts
- Salt to taste
- Freshly ground black pepper to taste
- 1/2 lime, cut into wedges

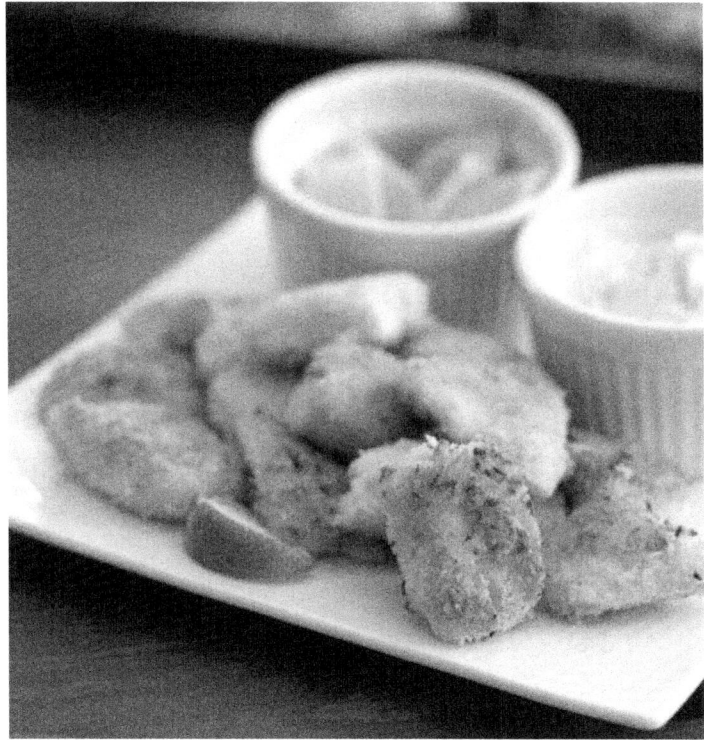

Directions:

1. In a skillet, warm the avocado oil at high heat. You want the oil to be about 1/2 inch deep, so adjust the amount of oil-based on the size of your pan.
2. Pat the fish to try using paper towels to take off any excess water.
3. In a small bowl, put and combine the eggs and mayonnaise.

- 1/4 cup dairy-free tartar sauce

Nutrition:

- Calories: 733
- Fat: 53 g
- Carbohydrates: 10 g
- Fiber: 6 g
- Net Carbohydrates: 4 g
- Protein: 54 g

4. In a medium mixing bowl, put and combine the almond flour, coconut, and macadamia nuts. Season with salt and pepper. Cut the mahi-mahi into nuggets.

5. Put the fish into the egg mixture then dredge in the dry mix. Press into the dry mixture so that "breading" sticks well on all sides.

6. Add the fish into the hot oil. It should sizzle when you add the nuggets. Cook for 2 minutes per side, until golden and crispy.

7. Place the cooked nuggets on a paper towel-lined plate and squirt the lime wedges and tartar sauce over them.

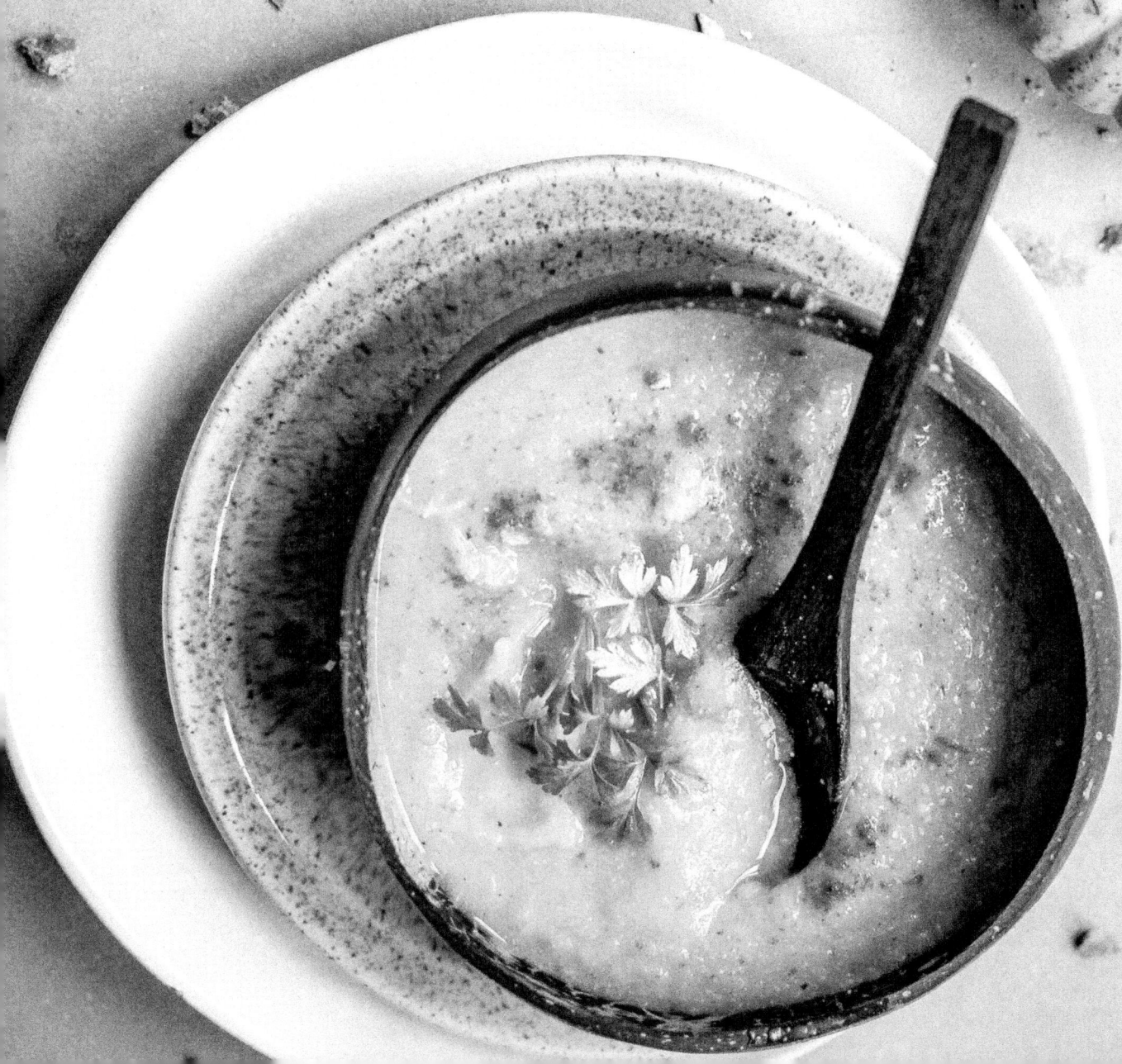

veggies
&
dips

36. Radish, Carrot and Cilantro Salad

Preparation time: 15 mins

Cooking time: 0 minutes

Servings: 2

Ingredients:

- 1 1/2 lb. carrots
- 1/4 cup cilantro
- 1 1/2 lb. radish
- 1/2 tsp. salt
- 6 onions
- 1/4 tsp. black pepper
- 3 tbsp. lemon juice
- 3 tbsp. orange juice
- 2 tbsp. olive oil

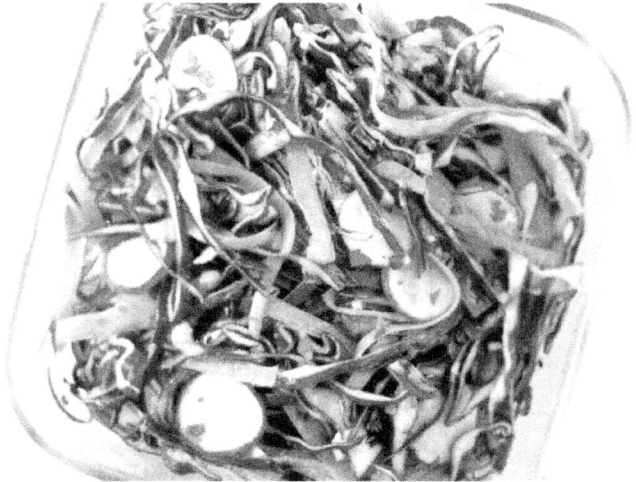

Directions:

1. Mix all the items until they merged properly.
2. Chill and serve.

Nutrition:

- Calories: 33
- Carbohydrates: 7 g
- Fat: 0 g
- Protein: 0 g

Preparation time: 10 mins

Cooking time: 5 minutes

Servings: 2

Ingredients:

- 2 loaves whole-wheat pita bread
- 3 tbsp. extra-virgin olive oil
- Salt and pepper to taste
- 1/2 tsp. sumac
- 5 pieces Roma tomatoes, chopped
- 5 pieces radishes stem removed, thinly sliced
- 5 pieces green onions, chopped
- 2 cups fresh parsley leaves stem removed, chopped
- 1-piece English cucumber, chopped

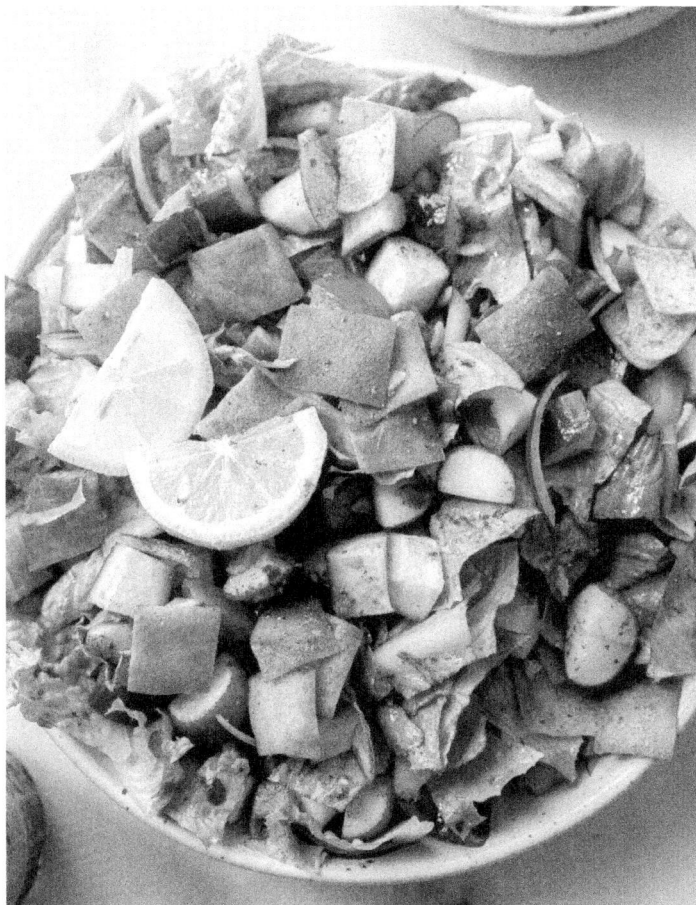

Directions:

1. In your toaster oven, toast the pita bread for 2 minutes until turning crisp, but is not browned.
2. Heat 3 tbsp. olive oil in a large frying pan. Cut the toasted pita bread into pieces and add them to the pan. Fry the broken pita

- 1 heart Romaine lettuce, chopped
- 1 cup fresh mint leaves, chopped (optional)

Dressing:

- Salt and pepper to taste
- 1 tsp. ground sumac or lemon zest
- 1 1/2 lime juice
- 1/3 cup extra-virgin olive oil
- 1/4 tsp. ground cinnamon
- 1/4 tsp. ground allspice

Nutrition:

- Calories: 478.8
- Fat: 18.1 g
- Fiber: 3.7 g
- Carbohydrates: 32.1 g
- Protein: 21.3 g

pieces for 3 minutes until browned, tossing frequently. Season the pita chips with salt, pepper, and sumac. Remove the seasoned pita chips from the heat and place them on paper towels to drain.

3. Combine the remainder of the salad ingredients in a large mixing bowl. Mix until fully combined.
4. Combine and whisk together all the dressing ingredients in a separate smaller mixing bowl. Mix well until fully combined.
5. Drizzle the lime-vinaigrette dressing over the salad. Toss gently to coat evenly.
6. Add the oil-drained pita chips and toss gently again until fully combined.

Preparation time: 10 minutes

Cooking time: 0 minutes

Servings: 2

Ingredients:

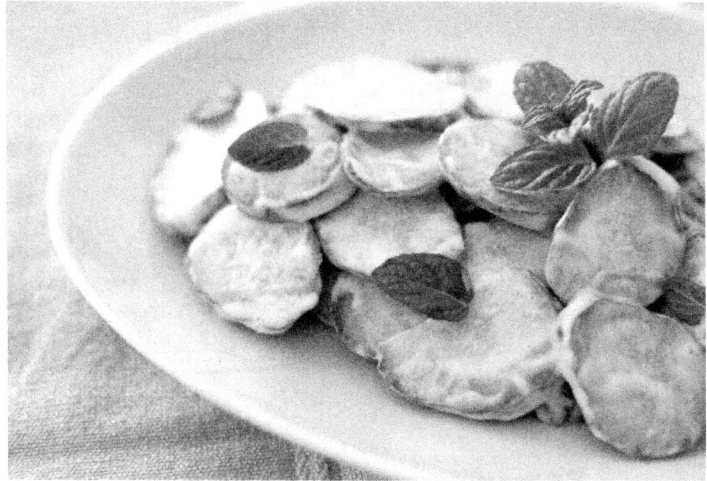

- 2 peeled and diced English cucumbers
- 1 1/2 tbsp. fresh garlic, crushed
- A pinch of salt
- 2 tsp. dried mint
- 1/8 tbsp. fresh dill, already minced
- 1-quart low-fat yogurt, plain

Directions:

1. In a small bowl, mix the dill, garlic, and salt.
2. Pour the yogurt in and mix well.
3. Add cucumber, mint and stir well
4. Put inside the refrigerator to chill, then serve.

Nutrition:

- Calories: 167
- Carbohydrates: 21 g
- Fat: 4 g
- Protein: 13 g

Preparation time: 10 mins

Cooking time: 0 mins

Servings: 2

Ingredients:

- 1/2 lb. white beans, cooked
- 1 onion, chopped
- 1 tbsp. lemon juice
- 7–8 cherry tomatoes, chopped
- 1 tbsp. oregano
- Ground pepper, to taste
- 2–3 tbsp. cilantro, chopped
- Salt, to taste

Nutrition:

- Calories: 345
- Fat: 27 g
- Carbohydrates: 67 g
- Protein: 21 g

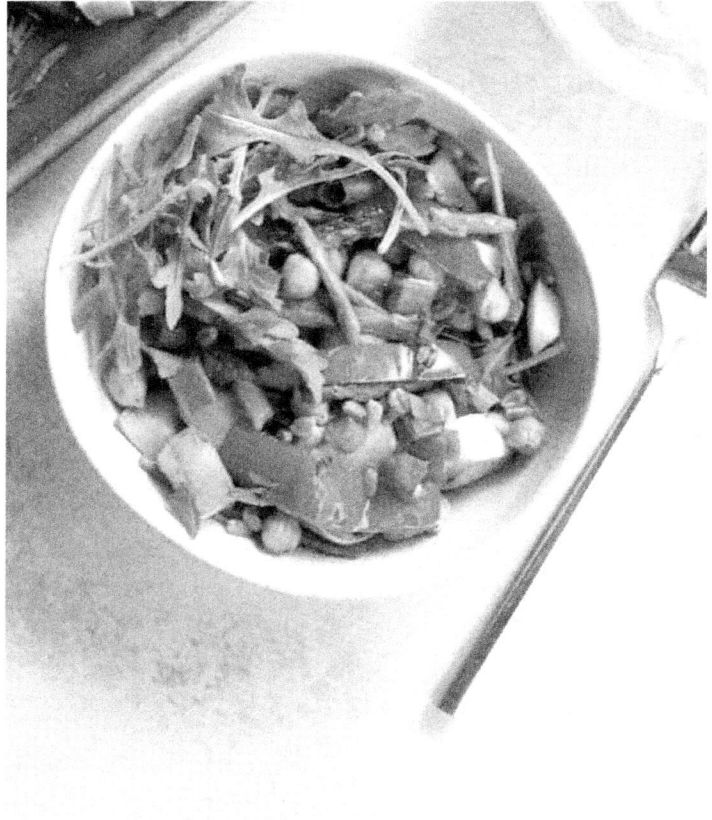

Directions:

1. In a large bowl combine white beans, onion, tomatoes, cilantro, oregano, salt, pepper, and lemon juice.
2. Add mixture to a serving dish.
3. Enjoy.

Preparation time: 5 Minutes

Cooking time: 10 Minutes

Servings: 4

Ingredients:

- 3 large green zucchinis
- 3 tbsp. extra-virgin olive oil
- 1 large onion, chopped
- 3 garlic cloves, minced
- 1 tsp. dried mint
- Salt to taste

Nutrition:

- Calories: 147
- Carbohydrates: 12 g
- Protein: 4 g

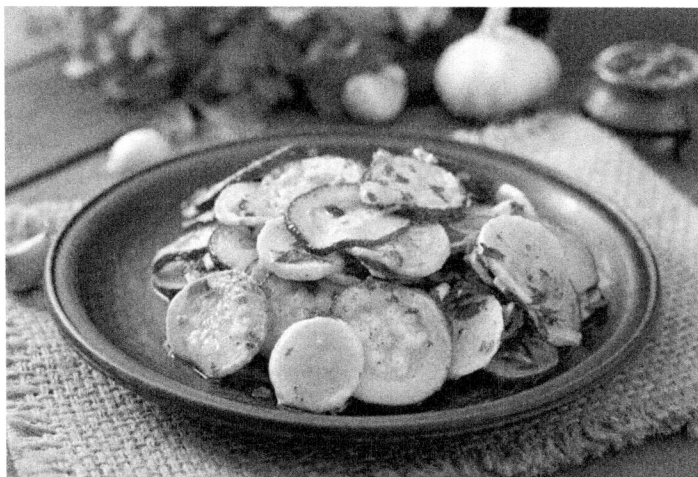

Directions:

1. Cut the zucchini into 1/2-inch cubes.
2. Using a huge skillet, place over medium heat, cook the olive oil, onions, and garlic for 3 minutes, stirring constantly.
3. Add the zucchini and salt to the skillet and toss to combine with the onions and garlic, cooking for 5 minutes.
4. Add the mint to the skillet, tossing to combine. Cook for another 2 minutes. Serve warm

Preparation time: 5 Minutes

Cooking time: 10 Minutes

Servings: 4

Ingredients:

- 1/4 cup extra-virgin olive oil
- 1 large onion, thinly sliced
- 3 garlic cloves, minced
- 6 (1 lb.) bags of baby spinach, washed
- 1 lemon, cut into wedges
- 1/2 tsp. salt.

Nutrition:

- Calories: 301
- Carbohydrates: 29 g
- Protein: 17 g

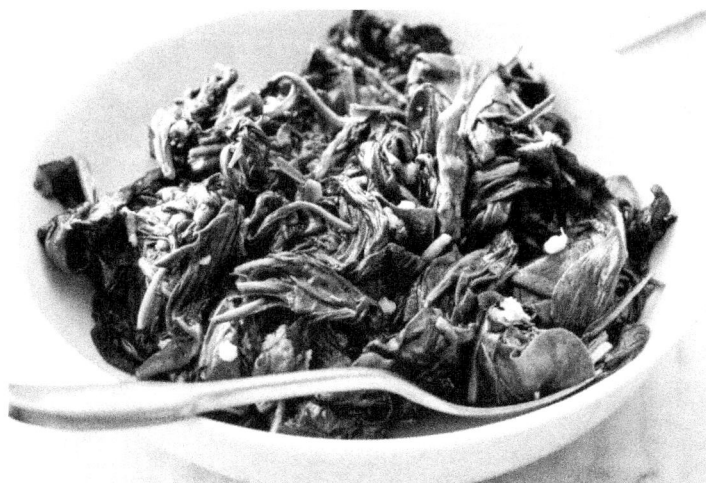

Directions:

1. Cook the olive oil, onion, and garlic in a large skillet for 2 minutes over medium heat.
2. Add one bag of spinach and 1/2 tsp. salt. Cover the skillet and let the spinach wilt for 30 seconds. Repeat (omitting the salt), adding 1 bag of spinach at a time.
3. Once all the spinach has been added, remove the cover and cook for 3 minutes, letting some of the moisture evaporate.
4. Serve warm with lemon juice over the top.

Preparation time: 5 minutes

Servings: 2

Ingredients:

- 1 cup sour cream (not plain)
- 2 tsp. dill pickle relish (not sweetened)
- 2 tbsp. white wine vinegar (not balsamic)
- 1 tsp. celery seed (to mellow the flavor, can substitute with garlic powder)

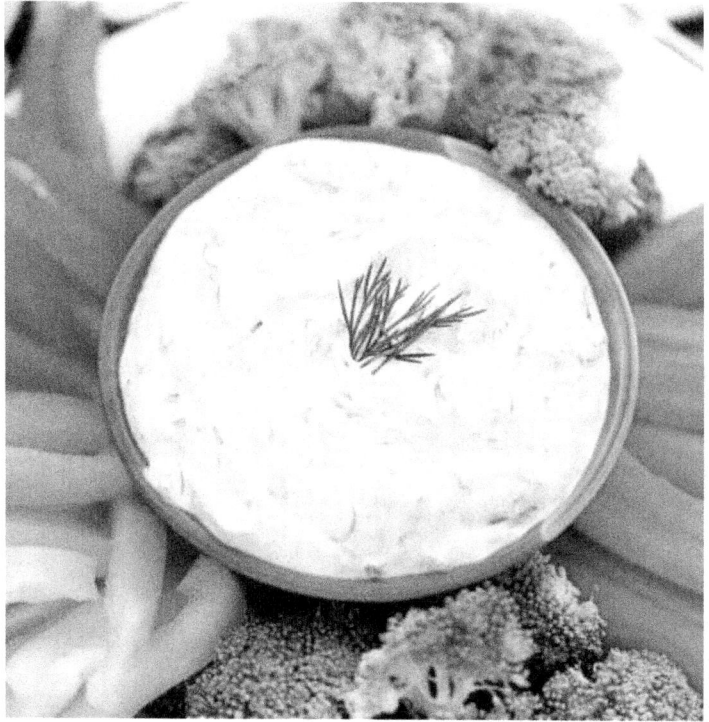

Nutrition:

- Calories: 43
- Fat: 4 g
- Carbohydrates: 0.9 g
- Fiber: 0.1 g
- Sugar: 0.5 g
- Protein: 1.2 g

Directions:

1. Place all ingredients in a small mixing bowl; whisk to combine. Chill for at least 30 minutes before serving. This dip tastes best when served within a few hours of its preparation so it is best to make a big batch and store it in the refrigerator until ready to serve.

Preparation time: 10 Mins

Cooking time: 5 Minutes

Servings: 4

Ingredients:

- 1 tomato, chopped
- 1 red onion, chopped
- 1 red bell pepper, deseeded and chopped
- 1 red chili, deseeded and chopped
- 4 garlic cloves, minced
- 2 tbsp. extra-virgin olive oil
- Juice of 1 lemon
- 1 tbsp. dried oregano
- 1 tbsp. smoked paprika
- 1 tsp. sea salt

Nutrition:

- Calories: 98
- Fat: 6.5 g
- Carbohydrates: 7.8 g
- Fiber: 3.0 g
- Sodium: 295 mg
- Protein: 1.0 g

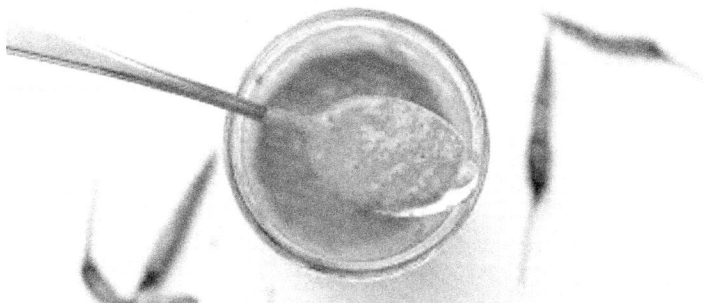

Directions:

1. Process all the fixings in a food processor or a blender until smooth.
2. Transfer the mixture to a small saucepan over medium-high heat and bring to a boil, stirring often.
3. Reduce the heat to medium and allow to simmer for 5 minutes until heated through.
4. You can store the sauce in an airtight container in the refrigerator for up to 5 days.

Preparation time: 10 mins

Servings: 2

Ingredients:

- 4 oz. Feta
- 1 cup plain Greek yogurt (not Greek style)
- 1 tbsp. fresh lemon juice (about 1 lemon)
- 2 garlic cloves, minced
- 1 jalapeño pepper, seeded and finely chopped (about 1 tsp.)
- 1/4 tsp. salt

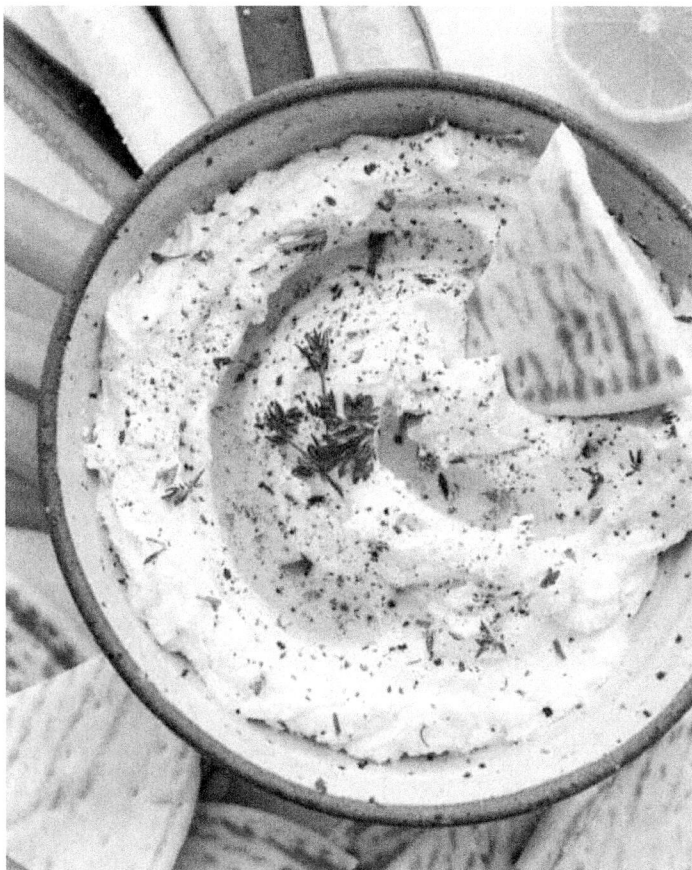

Nutrition:

- Calories: 116
- Fat: 8 g
- Carbohydrates: 2 g
- Fiber: 0 g
- Sugar: 1 g
- Protein: 9.5 g

Directions:

1. In a medium bowl, combine all ingredients. Cover and refrigerate for at least 30 minutes before serving. Best when served within several hours of preparation. Serve with pita wedges, crackers, or vegetables of choice.

Preparation time: 5 minutes

Servings: 2

Ingredients:

- 1 lb. radishes (about 1 1/2 cups), trimmed and very thinly sliced (about 3 cups)
- 2 garlic cloves, minced
- 1/4 cup sour cream or Greek yogurt (not plain)
- 1/4 cup mayonnaise or salad dressing (not salad dressing)
- 1/8 tsp. salt
- 1/2 cup shredded cheddar cheese (about 2 oz.)

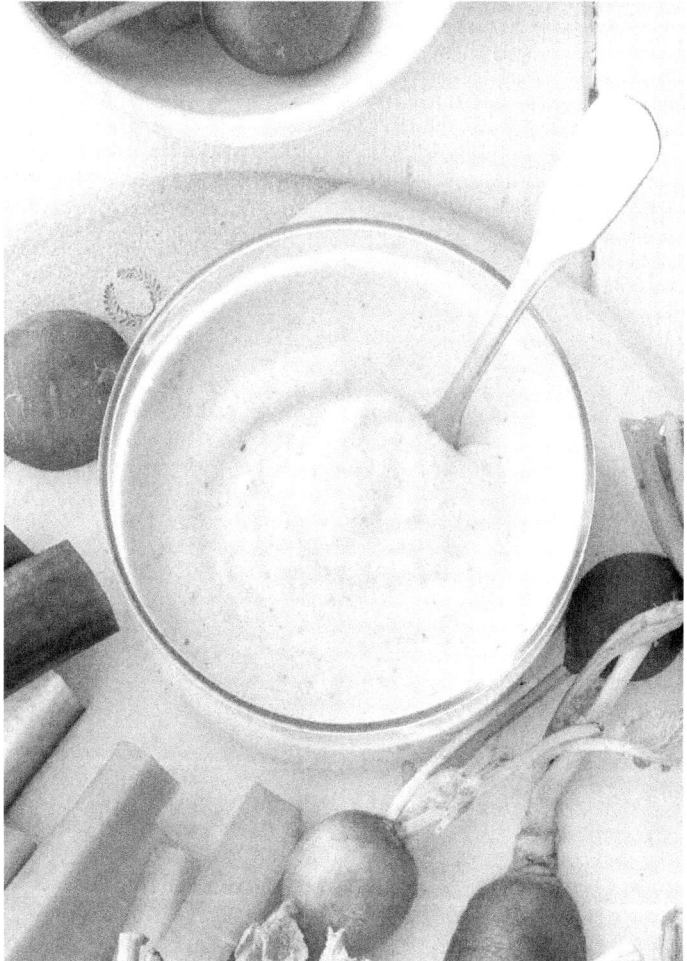

Nutrition:

- Calories: 83
- Fat: 4 g
- Carbohydrates: 2 g
- Fiber: 0.1 g
- Sugar: 0 g
- Protein: 3.2 g

Directions:

1. In a medium mixing bowl, combine radishes, garlic, sour cream, mayonnaise, salt, and cheddar cheese mix well. Serve immediately with pita wedges or crackers.

sweets
&
fruits

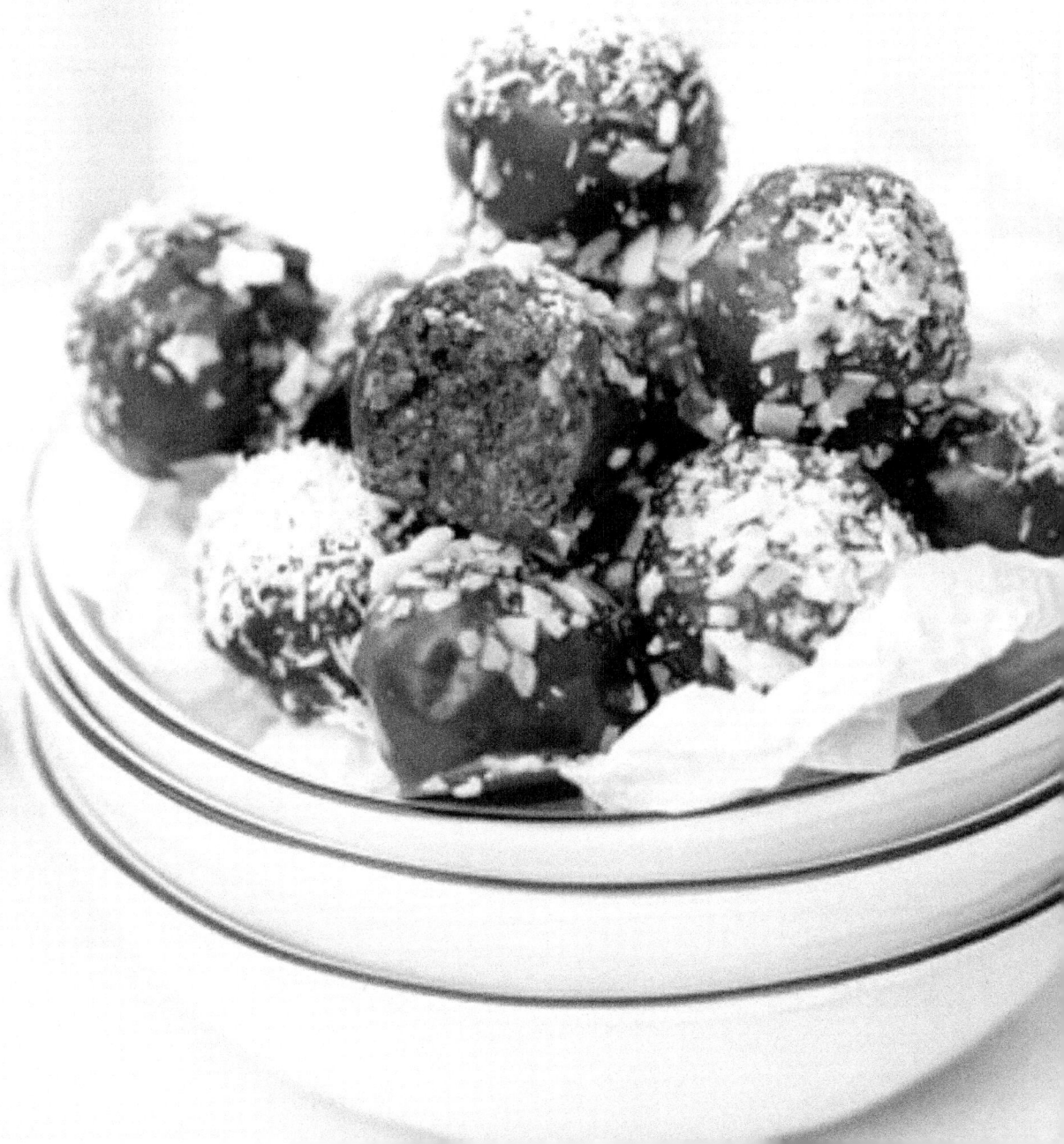

46. Delicious Coffee Ice Cream

Preparation time: 10 mins

Cooking time: 5 minutes

Servings: 1

Ingredients:

- 6 oz. coconut cream, frozen into ice cubes
- 1 ripe avocado, diced and frozen
- 1/2 cup coffee Expresso
- 2 tbsp. sweetener
- 1 tsp. vanilla extract
- 1 tbsp. water
- Coffee beans to taste

Nutrition:

- Calories: 596
- Carbohydrates: 20.5 g
- Fat: 61 g
- Protein: 6.3 g

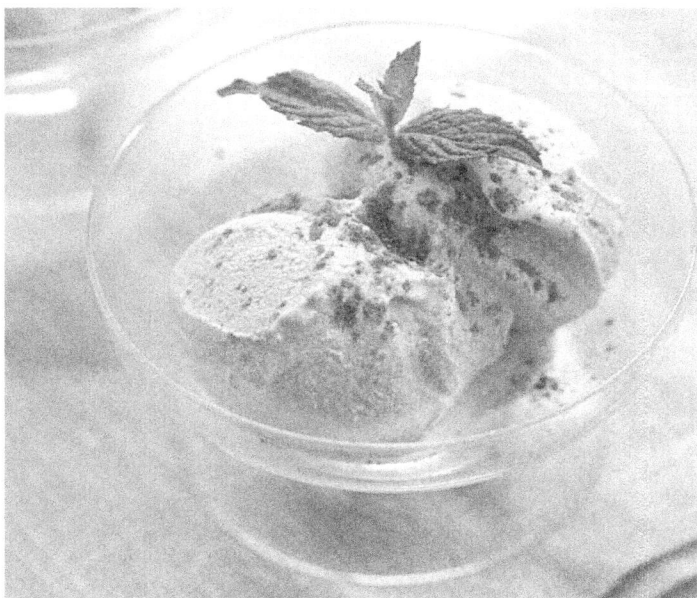

Directions:

1. Take out the frozen coconut cubes and avocado from the fridge. Slightly melt them for 5 to 10 minutes.
2. Add the sweetener, coffee expresso, and vanilla extract to the coconut avocado mix and whisk with an immersion blender until it becomes creamy (for about 1 minute). Pour in the water and blend for 30 seconds.
3. Top with coffee beans and enjoy!

Preparation time: 5 minutes

Cooking time: 5 minutes

Servings: 6

Ingredients:

- 2 tbsp. cacao powder
- 5 oz. hazelnuts, roasted and without shells
- 1 oz. unsalted butter
- 1/4 cup of coconut oil

Nutrition:

- Calories: 271
- Carbohydrates: 2 g
- Fat: 28 g
- Protein: 4 g

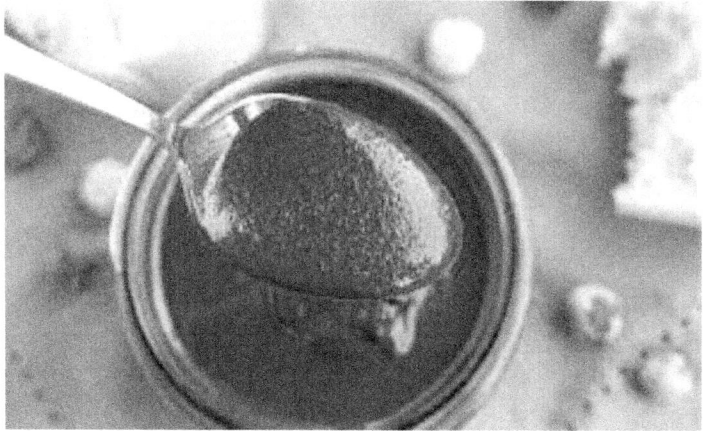

Directions:

1. Whisk all the spread ingredients with a blender.
2. Serve.

Preparation time: 5 minutes

Cooking time: 2 minutes

Servings: 4

Ingredients:

- 4 tbsp. almond flour
- 1 tsp. baking powder
- 4 tbsp. granulated erythritol
- 2 tbsp. cocoa powder
- 1/2 tsp. vanilla extract
- 2 pinches of salt
- 2 eggs beaten
- 3 tbsp. butter, melted
- 1 tsp. coconut oil, for greasing the mug
- 1/2 oz. sugar-free dark chocolate, chopped

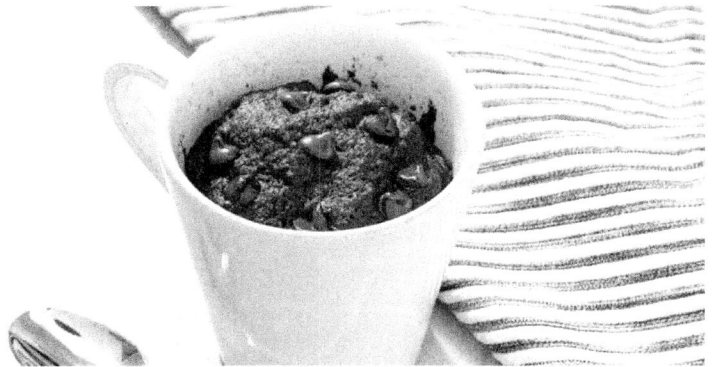

Directions:

1. Mix the dry ingredients in a separate bowl. Add the melted butter, beaten eggs, and chocolate to the bowl. Stir thoroughly.
2. Divide your dough into four pieces. Put these pieces in the greased mugs and put them in the microwave. Cook for 1–1 1/2 minutes (700 watts).
3. Let them cool for 1 minute and serve.

Nutrition:

- Calories: 208
- Carbohydrates: 2 g
- Fat: 19 g
- Protein: 5 g

Preparation time: 11 minutes

Cooking time: 5 minutes

Servings: 4

Ingredients:

- 6 egg yolks
- 1/2 cup unsweetened almond milk
- 1 tsp. vanilla extract
- 1/4 cup melted coconut oil
- Water

Nutrition:

- Calories: 215.38
- Carbohydrates: 1 g
- Fat: 21 g
- Protein: 4 g

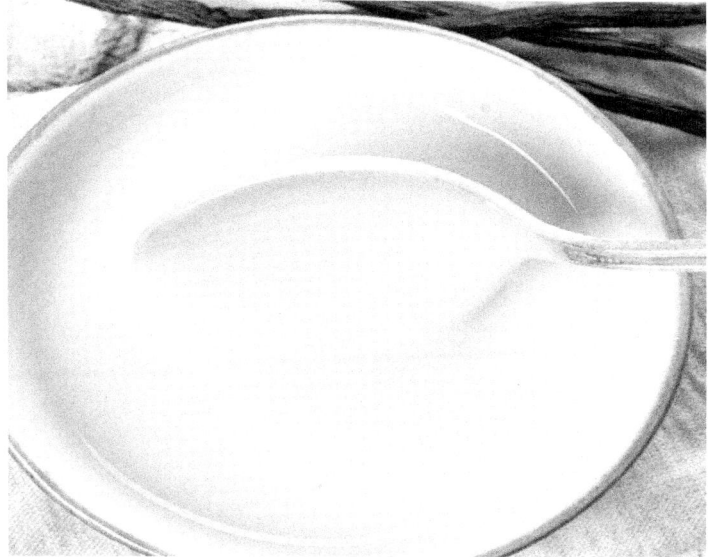

Directions:

1. Mix egg yolks, almond milk, and vanilla in a metal bowl.
2. Gradually stir in the melted coconut oil.
3. Boil water in a saucepan, place the mixing bowl over the saucepan.
4. Whisk the mixture constantly and vigorously until thickened for about 5 minutes.
5. Remover from the saucepan, serve hot or chill in the fridge.

Preparation time: 5 minutes

Cooking time: 5 minutes

Servings: 1

Ingredients:

- 3 large eggs
- 2 tbsp. sweetener
- 1 tsp. vanilla extract
- 1 tbsp. matcha powder
- 1 tbsp. butter
- 7 whole raspberries
- 1 tbsp. coconut oil
- 1 tbsp. unsweetened cocoa powder
- 1/4 cup whipped cream

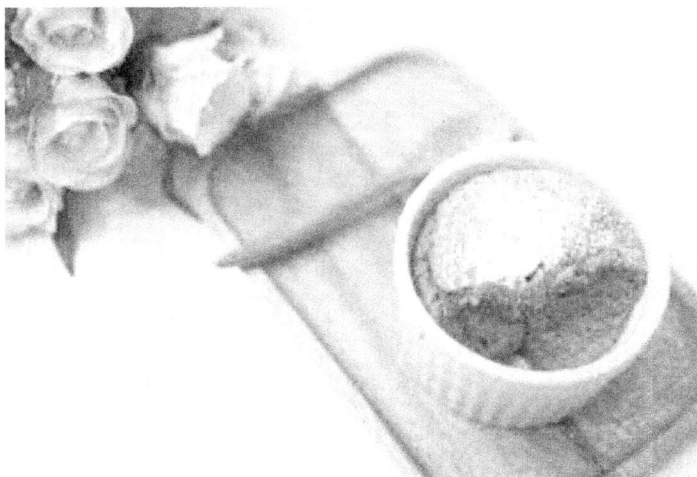

Directions:

1. Broil, then heat up a heavy-bottom pan over medium heat.
2. Whip the egg whites with 1 tablespoon of Swerve confectioners. Once the peaks form to add in the matcha powder, whisk again.
3. With a fork, break up the yolks. Mix in the vanilla, then adds a little amount of the whipped whites. Carefully fold the remaining whites into the yolk mixture.
4. Dissolve the butter in a pan, put the soufflé mixture in the pan. Reduce the heat to low and top with raspberries. Cook until the eggs double in size and set.

Nutrition:

- Calories: 578
- Fat: 50.91 g
- Carbohydrates: 5.06 g
- Protein: 20.95 g

5. Transfer the pan to the oven and keep an eye on it. Cook until golden browned.
6. Melt the coconut oil and combine with cocoa powder, whipped cream, and the remaining Swerve.
7. Drizzle the chocolate mixture across the top.

Preparation time: 5 minutes

Cooking time: 10 minutes

Servings: 2

Ingredients:

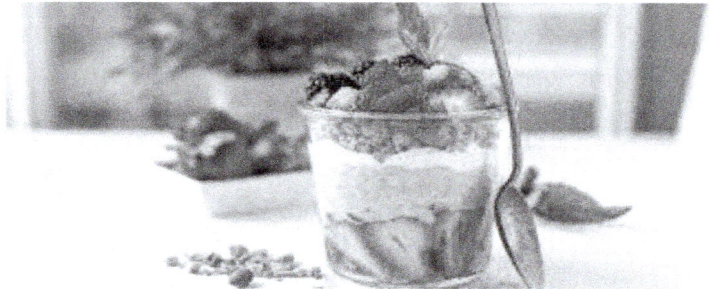

- 1/2 cup whole-grain rolled or quick-cooking oats (not instant)
- 1/2 cup walnut pieces
- 1 tsp. honey
- 1 cup sliced fresh strawberries
- 1 1/2 cups (12 oz.) vanilla low-fat Greek yogurt
- Fresh mint leaves for garnish

Nutrition:

- Calories: 385
- Fat: 17 g
- Carbohydrates: 35 g
- Protein: 21 g

Directions:

1. Preheat the oven to 300°F.
2. Spread the oats and walnuts in a single layer on a baking sheet
3. Toast the oats and nuts just until you begin to smell the nuts, 10 to 12 minutes. Remove the pan from the oven and set it aside.
4. In a small microwave-safe bowl, heat the honey just until warm, about 30 seconds. Add the strawberries and stir to coat.
5. Place 1 tablespoon of the strawberries in the bottom of each of 2 dessert dishes or 8 oz. glasses.
6. Add a portion of yogurt and then a portion of oats and repeat the layers until the containers are full, ending with the berries and mint leaves. Serve immediately or chill until ready to eat.

Preparation time: 10 mins

Cooking time: 5 minutes

Servings: 2

Ingredients:

- 2 cups fresh lychees, pitted and sliced
- 2 tbsp. honey
- Mint leaves for garnish

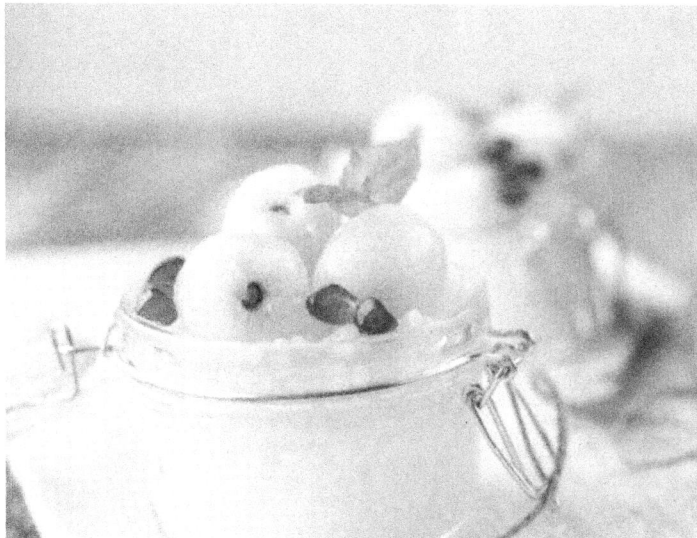

Nutrition:

- Calories: 151
- Carbohydrates: 38.9 g
- Fat: 0.4 g
- Protein: 0.7 g

Directions:

1. Place the lychee slices and honey in a food processor
2. Pulse until smooth.
3. Pour in a container and place inside the fridge for at least two hours.
4. Scoop the sorbet and serve with mint leaves.

Preparation time: 10 mins

Cooking time: 0 mins

Servings: 2

Ingredients:

- 1 orange, peeled and sliced
- 2 apples, pitted and diced
- 2 peaches, pitted and diced
- 1 cup seedless grapes
- 3/4 cup Greek-style yogurt, well-chilled
- 3 tbsp. honey

Nutrition:

- Calories: 250
- Fat: 0.7 g
- Carbohydrates: 60 g
- Protein: 6.4 g

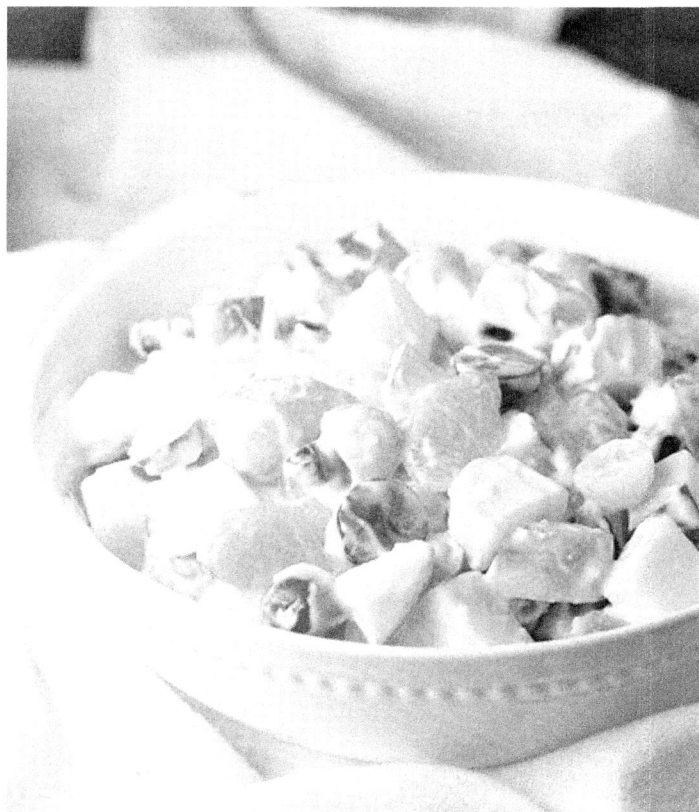

Directions:

1. Divide the fruits between dessert bowls.
2. Top with the yogurt. Add a few drizzles of honey to each serving and serve well-chilled.
3. Bon appétit!

Preparation time: 10 mins

Cooking time: 15 minutes

Servings: 2

Ingredients:

- 1 lb. strawberries (about 4–5 medium), washed and dried
- 2 scoops of whey protein powder (about 10 oz.)
- 2 cups water plus ice cubes (or almond milk)
- 1/4 cup coconut oil, melted (plus more for greasing the bowl)
- 1 cup fresh blueberries or frozen blueberries, thawed (about 2 oz.) or about 1 cup frozen blueberries (thawed as needed)
- 1/2 tsp. vanilla extract (optional)

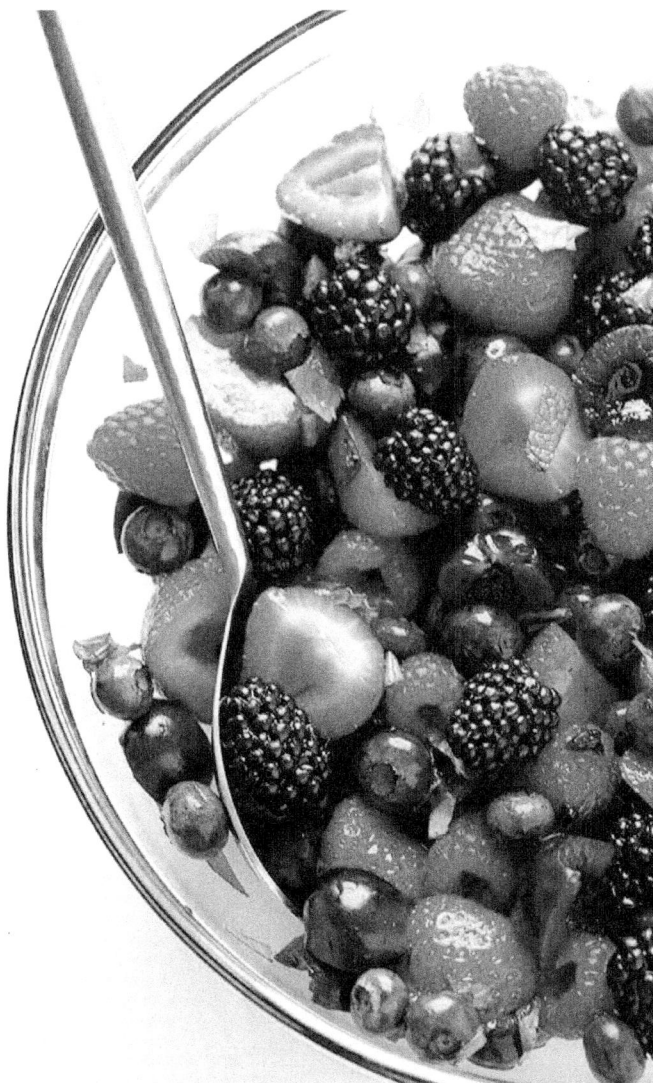

Directions:

1. Place berries on a large serving dish. Pour melted coconut oil over the berries and

- 1 cup Brown sugar
- 1 tbsp. Ginger
- 2 tbsp. Lemon juice

Nutrition:

- Calories: 162
- Fat: 14 g
- Carbohydrates: 2.9 g
- Fiber: 0.2 g
- Sugar: 1 g
- Protein: 9.2 g

drizzle with sugar-free syrup (if using) then sprinkle with protein powder.

2. Place four bowls over medium heat then add water, ice cubes (or almond milk), and whey protein powder to each bowl. Whisk frequently until the whey protein smooths out and is dissolved in the water/ice cubes. Add more ice cubes to each bowl as needed; bring to a simmer, stirring constantly until smooth and creamy (about 15 minutes).

3. Meanwhile, add brown sugar, ginger, lemon juice, vanilla extract, and blueberries into the blender; blend on a high setting until smooth (about 30 seconds). Pour into small glasses and serve immediately.

Preparation time: 10 minutes

Cooking time: 0 minutes

Servings: 2

Ingredients:

- 1/2 pineapple, diced
- 2 cups Greek-style yogurt, frozen
- 3 oz. almonds, slivered

Nutrition:

- Calories: 307
- Fat: 14.4 g
- Carbohydrates: 29.1 g
- Protein: 18 g

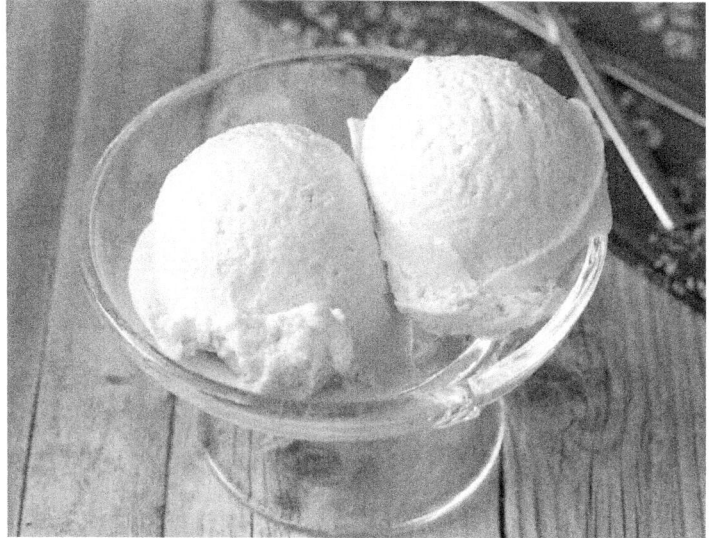

Directions:

1. Divide the pineapple between two dessert bowls. Spoon the yogurt over it.
2. Top with the slivered almonds.
3. Cover and place in your refrigerator until you're ready to serve. Bon appétit!

Chapter 6. Measurement Conversion

Volume Equivalents (Liquid)

Type	US Standard (oz.)	Metric
2 tbsp.	1 fl. oz.	30 mL
1/4 cup	2 fl. oz.	60 mL
1/2 cup	4 fl. oz.	120 mL
1 cup	8 fl. oz.	240 mL

Volume Equivalents (Dry)

Type	Metric
1/4 tsp.	1 mL
1/2 tsp.	2 mL
1 tsp.	5 mL
1 tbsp.	15 mL
1/4 cup	59 mL
1/2 cup	118 mL
1 cup	235 mL

Oven Temperatures

Fahrenheit (°F)	Celsius (°C)
250	120
300	150
325	165
350	180
375	190
400	200
425	220
450	230

WEEK		MONDAY	
MEAL			
	BREAKFAST		
	SNACK		
	LUNCH		

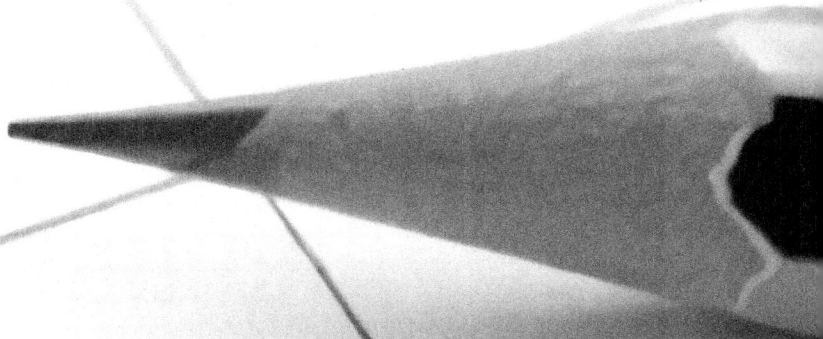

Chapter 7. 28 Days Meal Plan

Day	Breakfast	Lunch	Dinner	Desserts
1	Bacon and Avocado Omelet	Cilantro Chicken Breasts with Mayo-Avocado Sauce	Lamb Burgers with Tzatziki	Delicious Coffee Ice Cream
2	Keto Smoked Salmon with Avocado Slice	Sweet Garlic Chicken Skewers	Blackened Fish Tacos with Slaw	Chocolate Spread with Hazelnuts
3	Keto Cereal with Almond Milk and Walnuts	Lamb Burgers with Tzatziki	Thai Keto Tuna Salad Wrap	Chocolate Mug Muffins
4	Kale Fritters	Thai Keto Tuna Salad Wrap	Creamy Keto Fish Casserole	Keto and Dairy-Free Vanilla Custard
5	Cream Cheese Eggs	Keto Chinese Pork Stew with Cabbage	Coconut Mahi-Mahi Nuggets	Matcha Skillet Soufflé
6	Creamy Basil Baked Sausage	Lamb Sliders	Zingy Lemon Fish	Oat and Fruit Parfait
7	Strawberry Rhubarb Smoothie	Keto Zucchini Lasagna	Keto Seafood Chowder	Deliciously Cold Lychee Sorbet
8	Ricotta Cloud Pancakes	Blackened Fish Tacos with Slaw	Cilantro Chicken Breasts with Mayo-Avocado Sauce	Creamed Fruit Salad
9	Keto Cinnamon Coffee	Chicken Bacon Burger	Lamb Sliders	Strawberry, Blueberry, Lemon Juice, Ginger and Brown Sugar Salad
10	Keto Coconut Flake Balls	Zingy Lemon Fish	Keto Zucchini Lasagna	Greek Frozen Yogurt Dessert

11	Berry Smoothie	Garlic Steak Bite Salad with Tarragon Dressing	Salmon Skewers in Cured Ham	Delicious Coffee Ice Cream
12	Chocolate Banana Smoothie	Keto Pulled Pork with Roasted Tomato Salad	Cod Loin with Horseradish and Browned Butter	Chocolate Spread with Hazelnuts
13	Smoked Salmon and Poached Eggs on Toast	Lamb Burgers with Tzatziki	Garlic Steak Bite Salad with Tarragon Dressing	Chocolate Mug Muffins
14	Fruit Smoothie	Keto Harvest Pumpkin and Sausage Soup	Zingy Lemon Fish	Keto and Dairy-Free Vanilla Custard
15	Almond Coconut Egg Wraps	Salmon Skewers in Cured Ham	Chicken Bacon Burger	Matcha Skillet Soufflé
16	Bacon and Avocado Omelet	Keto Zucchini Lasagna	Lamb Sliders	Oat and Fruit Parfait
17	Keto Smoked Salmon with Avocado Slice	Creamy Keto Fish Casserole	Herby Fishcakes with Zucchini Salad	Deliciously Cold Lychee Sorbet
18	Keto Cereal with Almond Milk and Walnuts	Keto Seafood Chowder	Keto Pulled Pork with Roasted Tomato Salad	Creamed Fruit Salad
19	Kale Fritters	Herby Fishcakes with Zucchini Salad	Coconut Mahi-Mahi Nuggets	Strawberry, Blueberry, Lemon Juice, Ginger and Brown Sugar Salad
20	Cream Cheese Eggs	Stuffed Keto Mushrooms	Keto Chinese Pork Stew with Cabbage	Greek Frozen Yogurt Dessert

21	Creamy Basil Baked Sausage	Cilantro Chicken Breasts with Mayo-Avocado Sauce	Lamb Burgers with Tzatziki	Keto Coconut Flake Balls
22	Almond Coconut Egg Wraps	Sweet Garlic Chicken Skewers	Cod Loin with Horseradish and Browned Butter	Strawberry, Blueberry, Lemon Juice, Ginger and Brown Sugar Salad
23	Ricotta Cloud Pancakes	Coconut Mahi-Mahi Nuggets	Keto Harvest Pumpkin and Sausage Soup	Keto and Dairy-Free Vanilla Custard
24	Keto Cinnamon Coffee	Keto Chinese Pork Stew with Cabbage	Coconut Mahi-Mahi Nuggets	Creamed Fruit Salad
25	Keto Coconut Flake Balls	Keto Harvest Pumpkin and Sausage Soup	Salmon Skewers in Cured Ham	Deliciously Cold Lychee Sorbet
26	Chocolate Banana Smoothie	Garlic Steak Bite Salad with Tarragon Dressing	Stuffed Keto Mushrooms	Oat and Fruit Parfait
27	Smoked Salmon and Poached Eggs on Toast	Cod Loin with Horseradish and Browned Butter	Sweet Garlic Chicken Skewers	Chocolate Mug Muffins
28	Fruit Smoothie	Stuffed Keto Mushrooms	Cilantro Chicken Breasts with Mayo-Avocado Sauce	Chocolate Spread with Hazelnuts

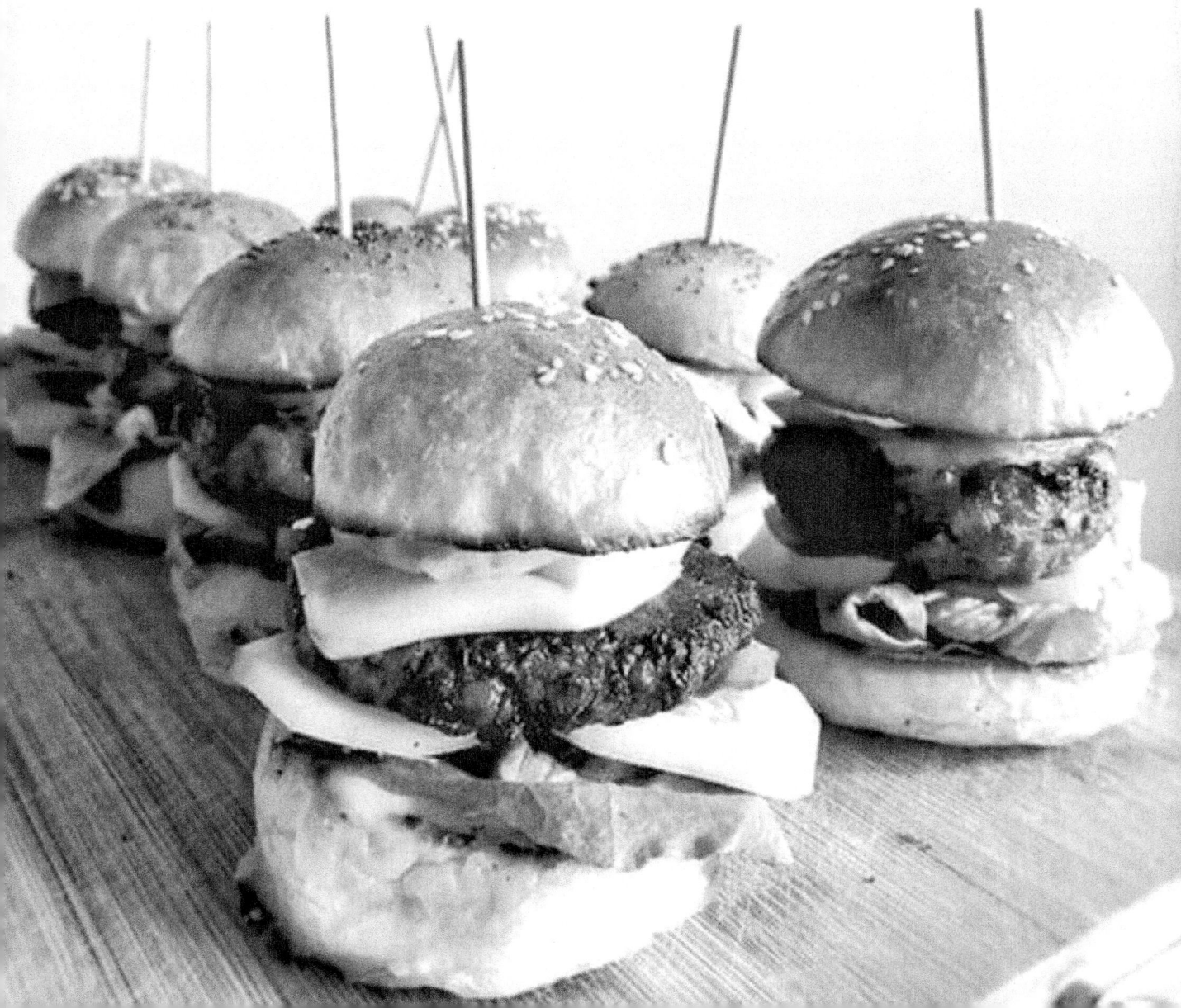

Conclusion

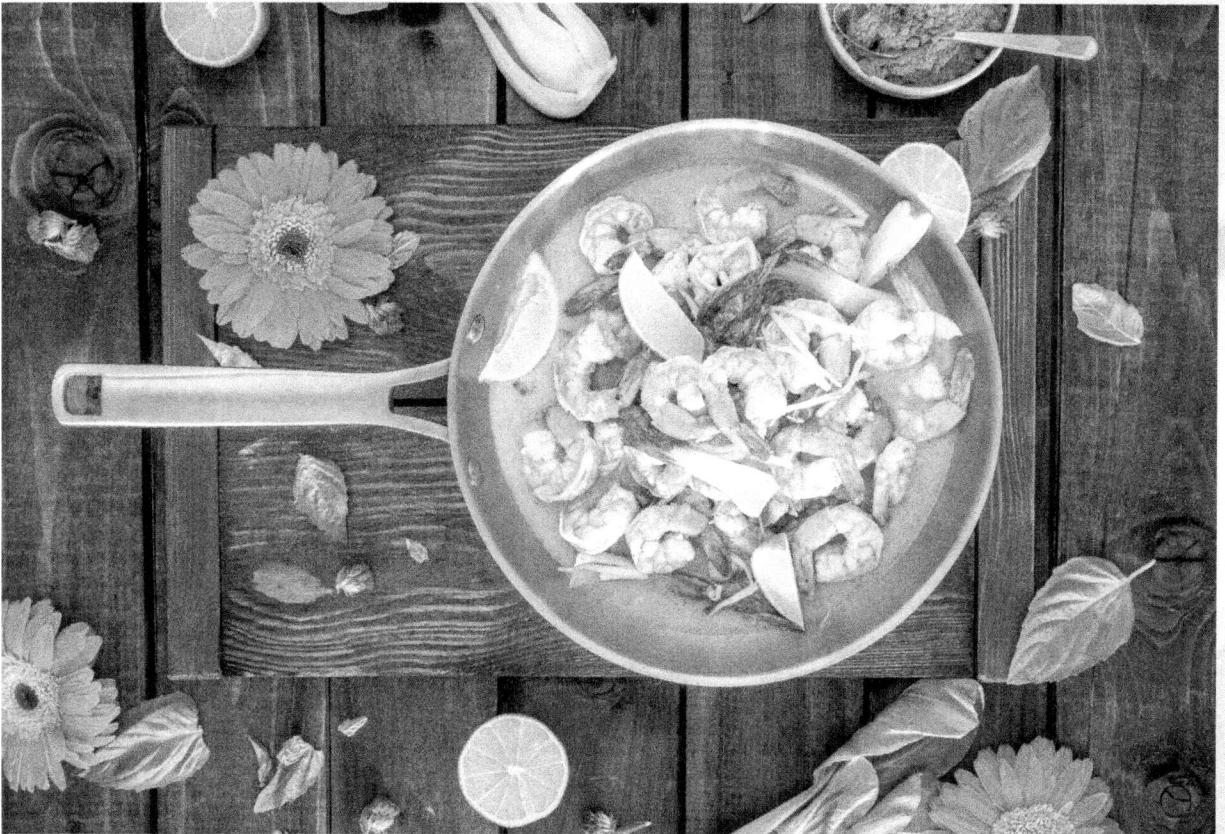

Ketogenic diet believes that by **minimizing your carbs** while maximizing the good fat in your system, making sure that you're getting **the protein you need** and help yourself aim with **daily physical exercises** becoming happier and healthier. In this book, we give you the information to know what this diet is all about, as well as describing the different types and areas that this diet will offer. Most people assume that there is only one way to do this and while there is one thing that the additional options share, there are minimum 4 different options you can choose from. Each one has its unique benefits, and you should know about each type to learn what would be best for your body, which is why we have described them in the book for you to have the best information possible when you begin this eating-training plan for yourself.

If you are faced with any difficult situations when following the keto diet, you should remind yourself of why you started the keto diet, to begin with, and what you are hoping to see from your diet health-wise or lifestyle-wise. No matter what your reason is for starting the keto diet plan**, you should focus** on that and try **to put difficult situations behind you.** If you are still having trouble coping with a certain situation, you can always ask for advice from one of your keto groups or like-minded friends. You never give up, face day by day improves must do and do it...even with the help of training plan.

The next step is to begin your **keto journey** and **start your new life**. Women and men over 50 need to take better care of themselves than ever before, so, if you have not made yourself your top priority before, **please do so now**. Now is the time for you to adopt the keto lifestyle and do everything in your power to make yourself better **physically and mentally**. Get your diet in order, begin a physical exercises routine, and start caring for you, the most crucial person in your life.

The aim of this guide is to drop you all the information you need to start your new healthy journey with the right foot. It's important to understand what you're getting into when and if you decide to start, all the valuable information you will discover here, you can use to your benefit and avoid the problems that you could face. You must stay healthy and make sure that your body can help you in everyday needs. Is always highly recommended, share your ideas and feelings with a nutritionist or your doctor to be sure that you are safe and that your body and your brain can handle this eating-training plan.

Use the knowledge to change your bad habits, learn how to prepare tasty meals for yourself, family, friends, or guests, improve how to heal your body and brain with daily physical exercises and enjoy life in the small things... as reading a book, finally.

P.S.

Your opinion on the book you just read is very important to me!

My goal is to know how to publish books of better quality in the future and to update and improve existing ones.

So, it would be great reading your feedback. Thank you

Best, Penny Craig

bubbly&Co press

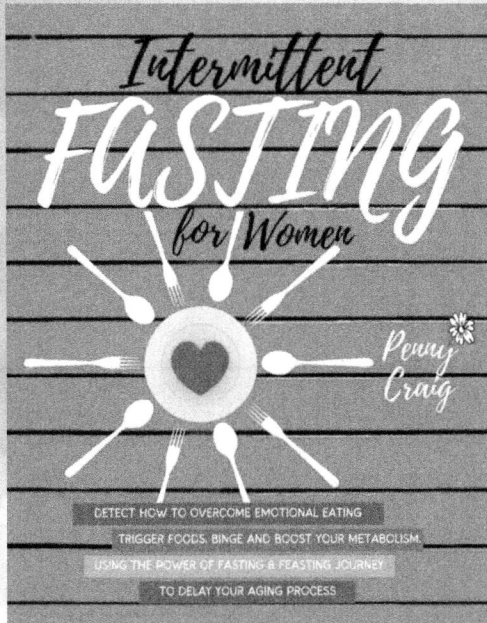

Intermittent FASTING for Women

Penny Craig

DETECT HOW TO OVERCOME EMOTIONAL EATING
TRIGGER FOODS, BINGE AND BOOST YOUR METABOLISM,
USING THE POWER OF FASTING & FEASTING JOURNEY
TO DELAY YOUR AGING PROCESS

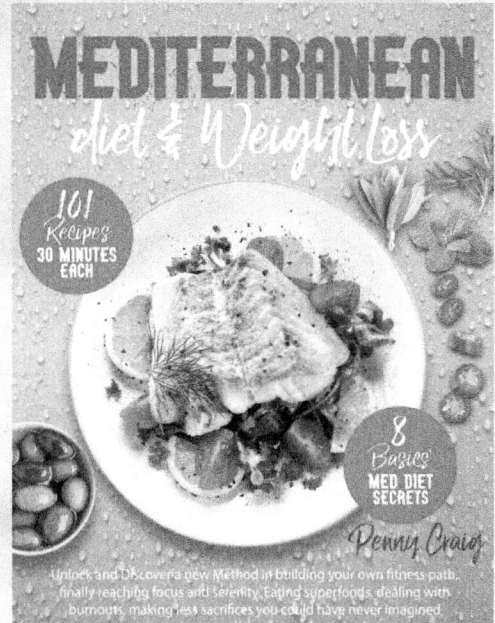

MEDITERRANEAN diet & Weight Loss

101 Recipes 30 MINUTES EACH

8 Basics MED DIET SECRETS

Penny Craig

Unlock and Discover a new Method in building your own fitness path, finally reaching focus and serenity. Eating superfoods, dealing with burnouts, making less sacrifices you could have never imagined.

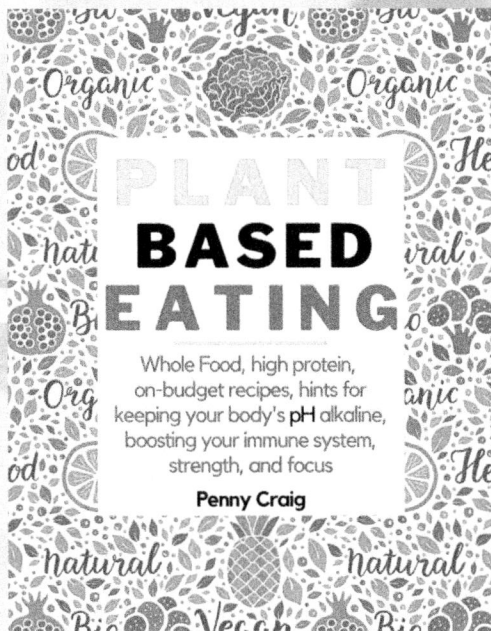

PLANT BASED EATING

Whole Food, high protein, on-budget recipes, hints for keeping your body's pH alkaline, boosting your immune system, strength, and focus

Penny Craig